# Orthopaedics

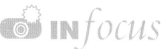

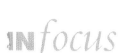
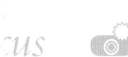

*Commissioning Editor:* Laurence Hunter
*Development Editor:* Siân Jarman
*Project Manager:* Anne Dickie/Anitha Rajarathnam
*Designer:* Charles Gray

# Orthopaedics and Rheumatology

## IN *f*ocus

AL Herrick MD, FRCP

Reader in Rheumatology and Consultant Rheumatologist, University of Manchester, Salford Royal NHS Foundation Trust, Salford, UK

## JG Andrew MB, ChB, FRCS, FRCS(Orth), MD

Consultant Orthopaedic Surgeon, Ysbyty Gwynedd, Bangor, North Wales, UK

## L Funk BSc, MSc, FRCS(Tr&Orth), FFSEM(UK)

Consultant Shoulder & Upper Limb Surgeon and Honorary Professor, Wrightington, Wigan & Leigh NHS Trust and University Salford, Salford, UK

## C Hutchinson BSc, MB, ChB, MD, FRCR, FFRRCSI

Senior Lecturer in Radiology, University of Manchester, Salford Royal NHS Foundation Trust, Salford, UK

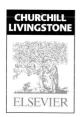

CHURCHILL LIVINGSTONE

ELSEVIER

EDINBURGH LONDON NEW YORK OXFORD PHILADELPHIA ST LOUIS SYDNEY TORONTO 2009

# CHURCHILL
# LIVINGSTONE
### ELSEVIER

© 2010, Elsevier Limited. All rights reserved.

No part of this publication may be reproduced or transmitted in any form or by any means, electronic or mechanical, including photocopying, recording, or any information storage and retrieval system, without permission in writing from the publisher. Permissions may be sought directly from Elsevier's Rights Department: phone: (+1) 215 239 3804 (US) or (+44) 1865 843830 (UK); fax: (+44) 1865 853333; e-mail: healthpermissions@elsevier.com. You may also complete your request on-line via the Elsevier website at http://www.elsevier.com/permissions.

First published 2010

ISBN: 9780443100864

**British Library Cataloguing in Publication Data**
A catalogue record for this book is available from the British Library

**Library of Congress Cataloging in Publication Data**
A catalog record for this book is available from the Library of Congress

**Notice**
Knowledge and best practice in this field are constantly changing. As new research and experience broaden our knowledge, changes in practice, treatment and drug therapy may become necessary or appropriate. Readers are advised to check the most current information provided (i) on procedures featured or (ii) by the manufacturer of each product to be administered, to verify the recommended dose or formula, the method and duration of administration, and contraindications. It is the responsibility of the practitioner, relying on their own experience and knowledge of the patient, to make diagnoses, to determine dosages and the best treatment for each individual patient, and to take all appropriate safety precautions. To the fullest extent of the law, neither the Publisher nor the Authors assumes any liability for any injury and/or damage to persons or property arising out or related to any use of the material contained in this book.

*The Publisher*

**ELSEVIER** your source for books, journals and multimedia in the health sciences
**www.elsevierhealth.com**

## Working together to grow
## libraries in developing countries

www.elsevier.com | www.bookaid.org | www.sabre.org

**ELSEVIER**    **BOOK AID** International    **Sabre Foundation**

The
publisher's
policy is to use
**paper manufactured
from sustainable forests**

Printed in China

# Acknowledgments

We are grateful to all those colleagues who have helped us by providing some of the illustrations for the textbook and to the staff of the Department of Medical Illustration at Salford Royal Hospital, who were responsible for many of the photographs.

Acknowledgments

# Contents

# 1 Musculoskeletal pain

Pain is one of the most common symptoms of musculoskeletal disease. The assessment and treatment of pain are crucial to the diagnosis and management of the different musculoskeletal conditions described in later sections.

*Clinical features*

Key points are:

1. Nociceptive versus neurogenic pain. *Nociceptive pain* is due to local tissue damage, for example, as a result of trauma or inflammation (Figs 1 & 2). It is often made worse by movement, and it responds to analgesics and anti-inflammatory drugs. It is usually localised to the site(s) of injury/inflammation but may be referred (or radiate) to other sites that share the same innervation as the injured part. *Neurogenic pain* is due to peripheral nerve or nerve root dysfunction. There is usually no sign of visible tissue damage. Its severity is out of proportion to apparent local tissue damage, and it is often unresponsive to analgesics. Neurogenic pain is frequently described as 'burning'. It can be associated with allodynia (a normally painless stimulus such as light touch is extremely painful).
2. Assessment of severity. This can be gauged by asking the patient if the pain disturbs sleep, about the number (and strength) of analgesics being taken, and by the functional limitations imposed.

*Investigation*

This will be dependent upon the nature of the underlying problem.

*Management*

Irrespective of its cause, pain must be promptly treated. The main challenges lie in the treatment of chronic pain and/or neurogenic pain (for which tricyclic antidepressants or anticonvulsants may be beneficial). Referral to a pain management team should be considered.

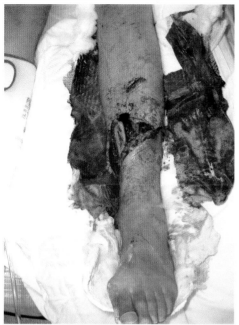

**Fig. 1** Nociceptive pain as a result of trauma.

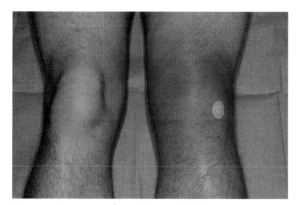

**Fig. 2** Inflammed area (prepatellar bursitis)—the knee was very painful especially anteriorly.

# Fibromyalgia

*Definition*

This is a common disorder characterised by diffuse, chronic, musculoskeletal pain. It can be primary, or coexist with other musculoskeletal diseases such as rheumatoid arthritis.

*Clinical features*

Patients complain of generalised pain and 'nonrestorative' sleep. For the diagnosis to be made, at least 11 of the following 18 points (in 9 pairs, right and left) should be tender (Fig. 3):

- Occiput (at the suboccipital muscle insertion)
- Low cervical (anterior aspect of the intertransverse spaces at C5–C7)
- Trapezius (midpoint of the upper border)
- Supraspinatus (at origin, above the scapula spine)
- Second rib (at the second costochondral junctions)
- Lateral epicondyle (2 cm distal to epicondyle)
- Gluteal (upper outer quadrant of buttock)
- Greater trochanter
- Knee (medial fat pad)

*Investigations*

These are performed to exclude other disorders. All blood tests should be normal.

*Management*

This is often difficult. Patients should be encouraged to keep active. Some patients benefit from low-dose antidepressants. Many patients have persisting severe disability and work incapacity.

# Reflex sympathetic dystrophy (Complex regional pain syndrome (CRPS) type 1)

CRPS is usually triggered by a preceding noxious event, for example an injury. Patients experience severe, persistent pain, which is neurogenic, usually beginning in an extremity but then extending proximally, and disproportionate to the inciting event. Swelling and changes in colour, temperature, and sweating are common (Fig. 4). Some patients go on to develop dystrophic change and contracture (Fig. 5). Radiographs show patchy osteoporosis. Treatment is difficult and is best delivered by a skilled multidisciplinary team. It is likely that early mobilisation after injury/surgery will reduce the risk of development of CRPS.

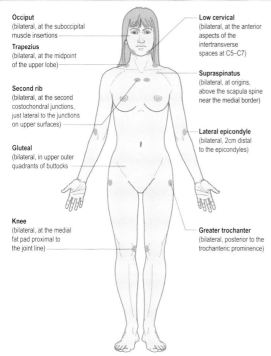

Occiput
(bilateral, at the suboccipital
muscle insertions

Trapezius
(bilateral, at the midpoint
of the upper lobe)

Second rib
(bilateral, at the second
costochondral junctions,
just lateral to the junctions
on upper surfaces)

Gluteal
(bilateral, in upper outer
quadrants of buttocks

Knee
(bilateral, at the medial
fat pad proximal to
the joint line)

Low cervical
(bilateral, at the anterior
aspects of the
intertransverse
spaces at C5–C7)

Supraspinatus
(bilateral, at origins,
above the scapula spine
near the medial border)

Lateral epicondyle
(bilateral, 2cm distal
to the epicondyles)

Greater trochanter
(bilateral, posterior to the
trochanteric prominence)

**Fig. 3** Checking tender points. (Reproduced with permission from Andrew JG, Herrick AL, Marsh DR. Musculoskeletal Medicine and Surgery. Elsevier-Churchill Livingstone, Edinburgh, 2000.)

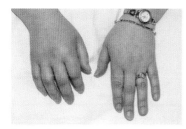

**Fig. 4** CRPS—the right hand is swollen and mottled and the fingers are held flexed.

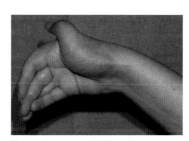

**Fig. 5** Late-stage CRPS with contracture and deformity.

Acute monoarticular arthritis is important as the differential diagnosis always includes septic arthritis—which may cause rapid and irreversible joint destruction if not diagnosed and treated.

## Septic arthritis

*Epidemiology*

Septic arthritis may occur at any age in either sex. It is particularly common in children including neonates, and is commoner in those with immune deficiency or previously damaged joints (thus especially frequent in diseases such as rheumatoid arthritis).

*Aetiology*

It is occasionally due to direct implantation (injury, surgery), but usually due to haematogenous spread.

*Clinical features*

### Symptoms

Patients have an onset of severe joint pain with inflammation and marked limitation of joint movement (Fig. 6). There may be systemic symptoms (malaise, fever).

### Signs

These typically include swelling, tenderness, and inflammation. There is usually severe limitation of joint movement (but not in neonates or the elderly). Function of the limb is severely restricted.

*Investigations*

Blood investigations are important (full blood count (FBC), erythrocyte sedimentation rate (ESR), C-reactive protein (CRP), blood cultures). Obtaining a bacteriological diagnosis is vital and requires aspiration of the joint under sterile conditions; aspirate is sent for microscopy, culture, and sensitivity. Consider whether TB is a possibility. X-rays are often normal but may show soft tissue swelling later and then destruction of joint and surrounding bone (Fig. 7).

*Management*

After aspiration, appropriate antibiotics are used. Staphylococci (especially *Staphylococcus aureus*) are the commonest organisms; agents such as flucloxacillin are often appropriate but this should be adjusted once the organisms are known. Prolonged treatment is often necessary. Joint lavage (with arthroscopy) may be required.

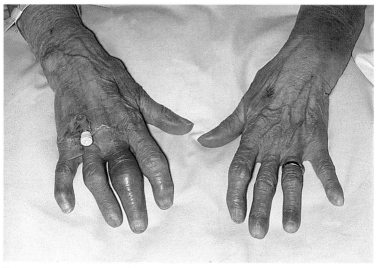

Fig. 6   Acute monoarthritis of the right middle proximal interphalangeal joint. This proved to be a septic arthritis.

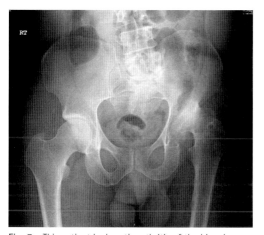

Fig. 7   This patient had septic arthritis of the hip when young—this has damaged the capital epiphysis and caused early osteoarthritis and affected growth of the femur.

# Gout and crystal arthropathy

Gout is a condition that causes episodic and recurrent acute arthritis.

*Epidemiology*

Gout is relatively common (1.5% of men over 30). Males are more frequently affected than females.

*Aetiology*

Crystal diseases involve acute precipitation of crystals in the synovial fluid causing a severe inflammatory reaction and consequent joint pain. The commonest is gout, where the incriminated crystal is urate (uric acid). Other crystal diseases include pyrophosphate arthropathy (pseudogout), which often causes calcification of meniscus and articular cartilage in the knee.

*Clinical features*

## Symptoms

Patients have a sudden onset of severe joint pain with inflammation and limitation of joint movement. In gout the first metatarsophalangeal (MTP) joint is often affected (Fig. 8), but other joints may also be involved. There may be a history of previous attacks; gout may be precipitated by some drugs (e.g. thiazide diuretics).

## Signs

Swelling and inflammation at the affected joint. There is restricted joint movement. In gout *tophi* are sometimes present (Fig. 9)—these are lumps of uric acid deposited in the soft tissues, usually at the elbow and hand.

*Investigations*

Exclude sepsis—FBC, ESR, CRP, aspiration of joint (microscopy, culture, and sensitivity). Confirm crystal disease—joint aspirate microscopy confirms crystals (negatively birefringent with polarised light in the case of urate) (Fig. 10). Serum urate level usually (not always) raised with gout.

*Management*

Acute crystal disease—nonsteroidal anti-inflammatory drugs (NSAIDs), analgesia. Occasionally colchicine is used for acute gout. In recurrent gout, allopurinol or a uricosuric agent is used to reduce urate levels and reduce recurrences. Persistent recurrences of gout lead to joint damage and osteoarthritis and it is important to maintain control in the long term. Precipitating factors should be avoided when at all possible (e.g. excess alcohol).

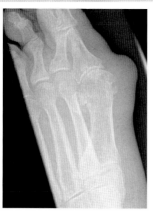

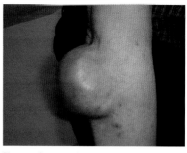

Fig. 9   Gouty tophus at elbow.

Fig. 8   First metatarsophalangeal joint showing consequences of inflammation due to gout. Note the periarticular position of the erosions and the amount of overlying soft tissue swelling.

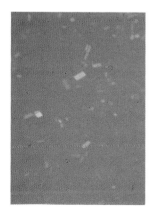 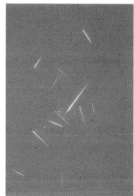

Fig. 10   Pyrophosphate (left) and urate (right) crystals in synovial fluid viewed under polarising light. (Reproduced with permission from Andrew JG, Herrick AL, Marsh DR. Musculoskeletal Medicine and Surgery. Elsevier-Churchill Livingstone, Edinburgh, 2000.)

Rheumatoid arthritis is the most common form of chronic polyarthritis (arthritis of several joints). The main clinical feature is synovitis (inflammation of the synovium). Joint involvement is usually symmetrical, and typically the small joint of the hands and feet are first affected, with the arthritis then extending proximally. All synovial joints can be affected. The clinical course is variable, with exacerbations and remissions. Some prefer the term 'rheumatoid disease' because this can be a multisystem disease with a variety of extra-articular features. Rarely internal organ involvement can be life-threatening.

*Epidemiology*

The prevalence in the UK is approximately 1%. It is 2–3 times more common in women than in men. Mortality is increased in patients with rheumatoid arthritis, with considerable recent interest in the increased mortality from cardiovascular disease.

*Aetiology*

This is unknown, but is almost certainly multifactorial involving both genetic and environmental factors. Increased understanding of the molecular and cellular pathology is driving new approaches to treatment, for example, with biological agents targeting tumour necrosis factor (TNF) alpha.

*Clinical features*

## Symptoms

The main symptoms of joint inflammation are pain, stiffness (especially in the morning or after inactivity), swelling, and symptoms related to loss of function.

## Signs

The main signs of joint inflammation are swelling (due to soft tissue thickening and/or effusion), tenderness, and pain on movement. Later in the disease deformity occurs. A key point is to distinguish between active disease (synovitis but possibly little or no deformity) and 'burnt-out', inactive disease, because this has important management implications (Figs 11 & 12).

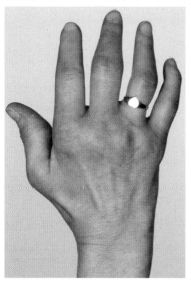

**Fig. 11**  Active rheumatoid arthritis—the metacarpophalangeal joints (especially index and middle) and proximal interphalangeal joints (especially middle and ring) are swollen. There is wasting of the dorsal interossei. There is an early Z-thumb, but otherwise little deformity.

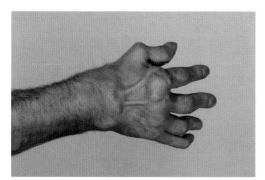

**Fig. 12**  More advanced changes of rheumatoid arthritis. In addition to evidence of active synovitis (affecting especially the index metacarpophalangeal joint and the wrists, where there is swelling that looks 'boggy') there is also obvious deformity (metacarpophalangeal subluxation, boutonnière deformities of the middle and ring fingers and a Z-thumb). Again there is marked wasting of the interossei.

## Hands

In early disease, spindling of the fingers occurs as a result of synovitis of the proximal interphalangeal (PIP) joints. Synovitis can affect not only the PIP, metacarpophalangeal (MCP), and wrist joints, but also the tendon sheaths of the fingers and wrist. Synovitis of the wrist flexors can lead to carpal tunnel syndrome. Rupture of the finger extensor tendons can occur. As the disease progresses, a number of typical deformities can develop:

* Ulnar deviation and flexion at the MCP joints
* Boutonnière deformity (flexion at the PIP joint and extension at the distal interphalangeal (DIP) joint; see Fig. 12)
* Swan-neck deformity (hyperextension at the PIP joint and flexion at the DIP joint; Fig. 13a,b)
* Z-thumb (flexion at the MCP joint and hyperextension at the interphalangeal (IP) joint)
* Dorsal subluxation of the ulnar head

## Feet

Metatarsophalangeal (MTP) subluxation is common and is a major cause of disability. Callosities and ulcers can occur beneath the metatarsal heads (Fig. 14a,b). Hallux valgus is common.

## Other joints

All synovial joints can be affected by rheumatoid arthritis, with signs of joint inflammation and/or deformity. Hip involvement is usually a late manifestation, but can be severe with marked restriction of movement. Knee involvement can be associated with popliteal cysts, which may rupture ('ruptured Baker's cyst'); this may be misdiagnosed as a deep venous thrombosis. Cervical spine involvement is common, especially subluxation at the atlantoaxial level, and neck movements may be restricted and painful; at worst, cervical spine instability may lead to cord compression.

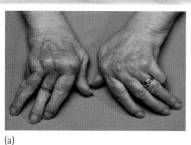 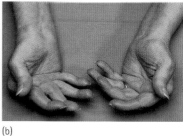

(a)　　　　　　　　　　　　(b)

**Fig. 13** Ulnar deviation and swan-neck deformities (a) dorsal and (b) palmar views in rheumatoid arthritis. The swan-neck deformities (affecting right index, middle, and little fingers) are best seen on the palmar view.

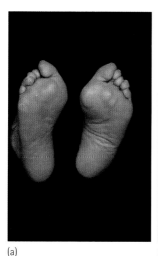 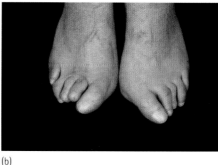

(a)　　　　　　　　　　　　(b)

**Fig. 14** Rheumatoid feet (a) plantar view showing MTP subluxation with overlying callosities and hallux valgus and (b) dorsal view showing flexion at the PIP joints with overlying pressure points. There are surgical scars on the right great, 2nd, and 3rd toes.

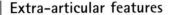

## Extra-articular features

### Rheumatoid nodules

The classic lesion of rheumatoid arthritis is the rheumatoid nodule, which typically occurs over pressure points such as the olecranon (Fig. 15). Nodules can ulcerate.

### Signs of vasculitis

Patients with rheumatoid arthritis can develop vasculitis. Features may include nailfold infarcts, cutaneous ulceration, and vasculitis of internal organs.

### Internal organ involvement

Signs of internal organ involvement should always be looked for. These include basal crackles (found in interstitial fibrosis), splenomegaly (which occurs in Felty's syndrome = splenomegaly and neutropenia in a patient with rheumatoid arthritis), and signs of neurological involvement (including entrapment neuropathy, cervical myelopathy, and peripheral neuropathy).

## Investigations

### General

Patients with active disease usually have a normochromic normocytic anaemia and an acute phase response (high ESR and CRP). Approximately 75% of patients with rheumatoid arthritis will be seropositive for rheumatoid factor at some point in their disease course. Synovial fluid analysis will show an inflammatory pattern (raised white cell count) in active disease.

### Imaging

The earliest change on plain radiographs is soft tissue swelling. This is followed by periarticular osteopenia, loss of joint space, and bone erosion. Radiographs of the hands and feet are useful in staging of disease—if repeated after a certain time interval, progression of disease may be evident (Fig. 16a,b). Cervical spine instability can be demonstrated on flexion and extension views (Fig. 17a,b), which are mandatory before general anaesthesia. Magnetic resonance (MR) scanning is extremely useful in the assessment of the rheumatoid neck.

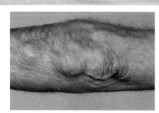
Fig. 15    Rheumatoid nodules at elbow.

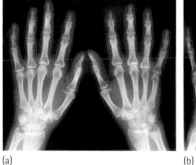
(a)

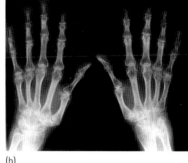
(b)

Fig. 16    X-ray of hands in a patient with rheumatoid arthritis in (a) 2000 and (b) 2004 showing erosive change of the carpus (with ankylosis of the right wrist) and small erosions of the MCP and PIP joints in the later film.

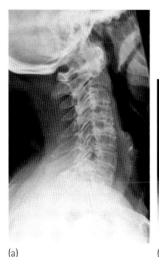
(a)

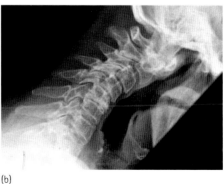
(b)

Fig. 17    Extension (a) and flexion (b) views of the cervical spine in a patient with rheumatoid arthritis—although there is no atlantoaxial instability there are forward slips of C2 on C3 and C4 on C5 in flexion, and erosive change especially at the C4/5 level.

### General principles

Effective management is multidisciplinary, and depends on a full assessment of disease activity and severity—management of early, active disease is very different from that of 'end-stage' disease with joint destruction but no ongoing inflammation. The key aspects are patient education, physiotherapy, occupational therapy, podiatry, drug therapy, and surgery.

### Physiotherapy

Patients should be taught exercises to prevent joint deformity and strengthen muscles. Many benefit from hydrotherapy.

### Occupational therapy

Simple and more complicated aids minimise the effects of disability, and help the patient to remain independent. Splints (to rest and/or support the joint) may be recommended (Fig. 18).

### Podiatry

Treatment of callosities, prevention of foot ulcers, and provision of suitable footwear (often with a moulded orthotic/insole) all help to minimise pain on walking (Fig. 19a,b).

### Drug treatment

Some drugs control symptoms (e.g. nonsteroidal anti-inflammatory drugs), others modify disease activity ('disease-modifying drugs', e.g. methotrexate). Disease-modifying therapy should be commenced early, before irreversible joint damage has occurred. While oral corticosteroids are highly effective in controlling inflammation, they have considerable toxicity, especially when used long term (e.g. osteoporosis). Intra-articular steroids suppress inflammation in individual joints. New biological therapies including anti-TNF therapies are now available for patients with active disease unresponsive to other drugs.

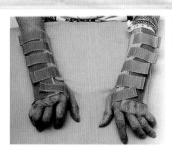

Fig. 18 Working splint. (Reproduced with permission from Andrew JG, Herrick AL, Marsh DR. Musculoskeletal Medicine and Surgery. Elsevier-Churchill Livingstone, Edinburgh, 2000.)

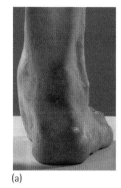

(a)

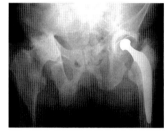

Fig. 20 Left-sided total hip replacement in a patient with rheumatoid arthritis and secondary osteoarthritis. On the right there are 'degenerative' changes with medial migration of the femoral head (more in keeping with rheumatoid arthritis than osteoarthritis).

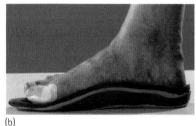

(b)

Fig. 19 (a) The foot of a patient with rheumatoid arthritis with flattening of the longitudinal arch. A moulded insole (b) makes walking much more comfortable.

## Surgery

Many patients will require a series of operations during the course of their disease and it is important that the order/timing is carefully planned. Commonly performed operations include MCP joint replacement, forefoot arthroplasty (excision of the lesser metatarsal heads), and knee, hip, elbow and shoulder replacements (Fig. 20).

Psoriatic arthritis is one of the seronegative spondyloarthropathies ('seronegative' because patients are seronegative for rheumatoid factor). Others are ankylosing spondylitis, reactive arthritis, and arthritis associated with inflammatory bowel disease (enteropathic arthritis). These conditions share certain clinical manifestations— enthesopathy (abnormality at the site of ligament or articular capsule insertion into bone) is a characteristic feature, as well as synovitis. Both peripheral joint and axial skeletal involvement may occur, and extra-articular features (including uveitis). There are different forms of psoriatic arthritis (one form is clinically indistinguishable from rheumatoid).

*Epidemiology*

Approximately 1% of the UK population have psoriasis. Of these, approximately 5% have psoriatic arthritis. Equal numbers of males and females are affected.

*Aetiology*

This is not known but as with rheumatoid arthritis is likely to be multifactorial. HLA-B27 is thought to be a susceptibility factor for the spondyloarthropathies.

*Clinical features*

### Symptoms

These reflect the pattern of joint involvement with swelling, stiffness, and pain on movement.

*Signs*

These are of joint inflammation and/or enthesopathy (e.g. tenderness and swelling of the Achilles tendon in Achilles tendonitis). The DIP joints (rarely involved in rheumatoid) may be swollen and tender (Fig. 21). Dactylitis ('sausage digit') is typical of the spondyloarthropathies (Fig. 22). Characteristic skin and nail changes may be present (Fig. 23).

*Investigations*

Anaemia and an acute phase response are found in active disease. X-rays may show loss of joint space and erosion (Fig. 24).

*Management*

This is multidisciplinary. Management of the spondyloarthropathies is broadly similar to that of rheumatoid arthritis. Methotrexate is often used as a disease-modifying drug and is beneficial for both skin and joint psoriasis.

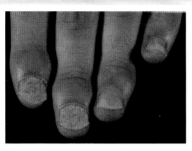

**Fig. 21** Psoriatic arthritis with DIP involvement and nail changes.

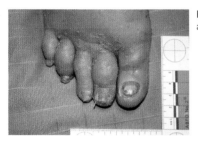

**Fig. 22** Dactylitis (2nd, 4th, and 5th toes) and psoriatic nail changes.

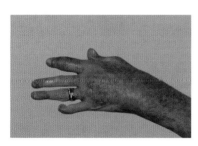

**Fig. 23** Advanced psoriatic arthritis with deformity (thumb, little finger) as well as dactylitis of index finger, nail, and skin changes.

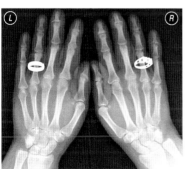

**Fig. 24** Erosive change especially at the DIP joints and left thumb IP joint in psoriatic arthritis.

# 8 Spondyloarthropathies: ankylosing spondylitis

Ankylosing spondylitis is primarily a disease of the axial skeleton (spine and sacroiliac joints).

*Epidemiology*

In white people, the prevalence is in the order of 0.5–1%. Over 90% of patients are HLA-B27 positive. The disease is approximately three times more common in men than in women. Onset is usually in young adults.

*Aetiology*

This is most likely to be multifactorial. The strong HLA-B27 association highlights the genetic component to the disease.

*Clinical features*

## Symptoms

The classic symptom is back pain in a young adult, worse with rest (e.g. first thing in the morning) and relieved with exercise. Symptoms of peripheral joint inflammation are less common, but can occur—in particular hip involvement can be severe and very symptomatic. Beware of the symptom of red eye, which suggests iritis.

## Signs

Lumbar and cervical spinal mobility can be reduced in all planes (Figs 25 & 26), and chest expansion reduced if the thoracic spine is involved. Tenderness over the sacroiliac joints may indicate sacroiliitis. Hip movements may be painful and limited.

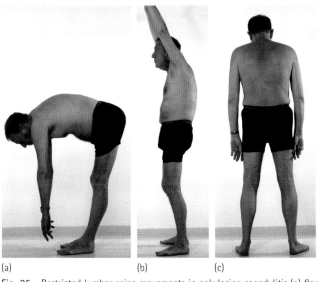

(a)                              (b)                    (c)

**Fig. 25** Restricted lumbar spine movements in ankylosing spondylitis (a) flexion (b) extension, and (c) lateral bending to the left.

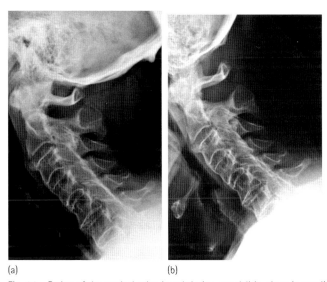

(a)                                        (b)

**Fig. 26** Fusion of the cervical spine in ankylosing spondylitis—there is very little movement between the extension (a) and flexion (b) views. Note the calcification in the anterior spinous ligament.

*Investigations*

The earliest abnormality on plain radiographs is erosion/sclerosis of the sacroiliac joints, which may later fuse (Fig. 27). In the lumbar spine, squaring of the vertebrae occurs and may be followed by formation of bony spurs called syndesmophytes (Fig. 28). In advanced disease, ossification of spinal ligaments causes a 'bamboo spine' appearance.

*Management*

Physiotherapy is the key point in management. All patients should have a home exercise programme. NSAIDs provide symptomatic relief. Anti-TNF drugs are now being used in patients with active disease.

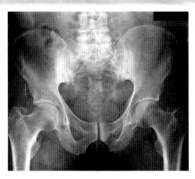

**Fig. 27** Sacroiliitis—sclerosis and erosion of the sacroiliac joints.

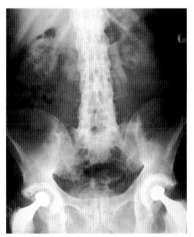

**Fig. 28** Advanced changes of ankylosing spondylitis—spinal fusion with syndesmophytes, fused sacroiliac joints, and bilateral total hip replacements.

## Reactive arthritis

Reactive arthritis develops in response to infection at a distant site (usually urogenital, gastrointestinal, or throat). The term 'Reiter's sydrome' is often used when the arthritis follows a sexually transmitted or diarrhoeal illness, the classic triad of clinical features being arthritis, conjunctivitis (Fig. 29), and urethritis. Most patients recover spontaneously, although some develop chronic disease. In the order of 70% to 80% of patients are HLA-B27 positive.

*Epidemiology*

Reactive arthritis is usually a disease of young adults. Males and females are equally affected.

*Clinical features*

These are similar to those of the other spondyloarthopathies. In the spondyloarthropathies (with the exception of psoriatic arthritis) peripheral joint involvement tends to be predominantly lower limb and asymmetrical. Patients presenting with joint inflammation should always be asked about preceding infections. Mucocutaneous lesions including balanitis and conjunctivitis are common. A rash of the feet called 'keratoderma blenorrhagica' can occur (Fig. 30). This is clinically indistinguishable from pustular psoriasis.

*Management*

Antibiotic treatment is indicated if an organism is isolated. Disease-modifying drugs are seldom required.

## Enteropathic arthritis

*Introduction*

Enteropathic arthritis is associated with inflammatory bowel disease (Crohn's disease or ulcerative colitis).

*Epidemiology*

Between 2% and 20% of patients with inflammatory bowel disease develop arthritis.

*Clinical features*

These are similar to those of the other spondyloarthopathies. Flares of peripheral arthritis often coincide with flares of the gut disease.

*Management*

Caution must be taken with nonsteroidal anti-inflammatory drugs. Sulfasalazine is often prescribed as a disease-modifying drug.

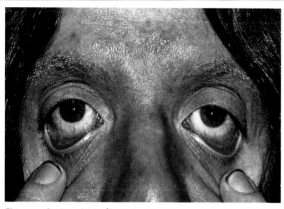

**Fig. 29** Conjunctivitis. (Reproduced with permission from Moll JMH, Rheumatology colour guide, 2e. Elsevier-Churchill Livingstone, Edinburgh, 1997.)

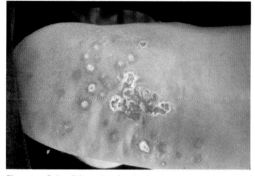

**Fig. 30** Sole of foot showing keratoderma blenorrhagica.

**Connective tissue diseases and vasculitides: general features**

The connective tissue diseases and vasculitides are multisystem diseases affecting connective tissues and blood vessels. Most are uncommon. However, they are important to recognise because they can be life-threatening. Most are inflammatory (the exception is systemic sclerosis, in which inflammation is less important than fibrosis and ischaemic atrophy) and all have systemic features. Most are associated with circulating autoantibodies.

The connective tissue diseases which will be considered specifically in later sections are:

- Systemic lupus erythematosus (SLE) and antiphospholipid syndrome
- Systemic sclerosis
- Inflammatory muscle disease
- Sjogren's syndrome
- The vasculitides (with brief mention of individual diseases)

It is important to realise that all these conditions overlap, and that certain general points can be made regarding aetiology, clinical features, investigation, and management. These general points will not be repeated in later sections.

*Aetiology*

Usually the aetiology is unknown, but is likely to be multifactorial and involve a combination of genetic and environmental factors.

*Clinical features and investigations*

These reflect the inflammatory, multisystem nature of this group of diseases. Features that should make one suspect a connective tissue disease include tiredness, malaise, weight loss, unexplained fever, joint or muscle inflammation, splinter haemorrhages, a vasculitic rash (Fig. 31), Raynaud's phenomenon, features consistent with internal organ ischaemia or with multisystem disease, anaemia, and an acute phase response (e.g. raised ESR or CRP). Many patients will be antinuclear antibody (ANA) positive (Fig. 32), and some will have disease-specific antibodies. Investigation of an individual patient will depend upon the likely pattern of internal organ involvement.

*Management*

This is multidisciplinary. Patients with active, severe disease may require corticosteroids and/or immunosuppressants.

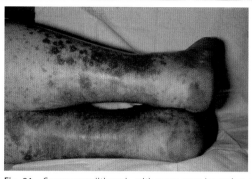

**Fig. 31** Severe vasculitic rash, with some areas becoming necrotic.

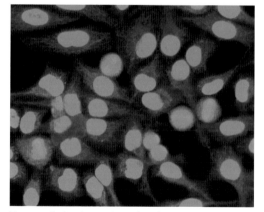

**Fig. 32** Antinuclear antibody (ANA)—homogeneous staining pattern on Hep2 cells. Courtesy of A. Moran.

Major internal organ involvement (renal, pulmonary, cardiac, neuropsychiatric, haematological) can be life-threatening. Some patients have an associated antiphospholipid syndrome, which is characterised clinically by thrombosis (either arterial or venous), pregnancy loss, and thrombocytopenia, and in the laboratory by the presence of anticardiolipin antibodies and/or lupus anticoagulant. Pregnancy may adversely affect SLE, and SLE may adversely affect pregnancy.

*Epidemiology*

Women are most commonly affected (female : male ratio is around 9 : 1) during their reproductive years. SLE is commoner in Asians and Afro-Caribbeans than in whites.

*Aetiology*

This is unknown. Certain drugs (e.g. hydralazine) can induce SLE.

*Clinical features*

Almost any clinical feature may be a result of SLE. Common features include tiredness, fever, photosensitivity (with a malar rash; Fig. 33), mouth ulcers, alopecia, Raynaud's phenomenon, secondary Sjogren's syndrome (dry eyes and mouth), and arthralgia/arthritis. Always consider the possibility of infection in the unwell patient with SLE (Fig. 34). Patients with SLE are at increased risk of atherosclerosis.

*Investigations*

Regular Dipstix testing of the urine (for blood and protein) may give an early pointer to renal disease. Anaemia (which may be haemolytic), leucopenia, and thrombocytopenia may all occur. More than 95% of patients are antinuclear antibody positive. Double-stranded DNA antibodies are highly specific for SLE and can be a useful measure of disease activity.

*Management*

Patients should wear strong sunblock when appropriate. Blood pressure should be carefully monitored and controlled. Many patients benefit from antimalarials. Steroids and/or immunosuppressant therapy are indicated in active, severe disease. Prepregnancy counselling is important in young women.

*Clinical course*

This is variable and depends on the degree of internal organ involvement.

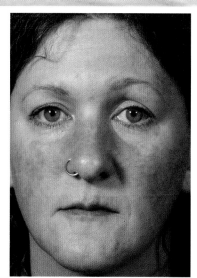

**Fig. 33** Malar 'butterfly' rash of SLE.

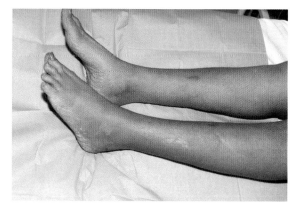

**Fig. 34** Monoarthritis of the left ankle in a patient with SLE, presumed septic. Patients with SLE are at increased risk of sepsis. The ankle is swollen and erythematous, and on palpation was warm and tender. Movement was very painful.

The main clinical features of systemic sclerosis are a result of fibrosis and/or ischaemia. Internal organ involvement (cardiorespiratory (including pulmonary hypertension), renal, gastrointestinal) can be life-threatening. There are two major subtypes, defined on the basis of the extent of the skin involvement—limited cutaneous (previously termed CREST—calcinosis (Fig. 35), Raynaud's phenomenon, oesophageal involvement, sclerodactyly, and telangiectases) and diffuse cutaneous. In diffuse cutaneous disease, skin changes extend proximally to involve proximal limb and/or trunk. The two subtypes have different natural histories, autoantibody associations, and prognoses.

*Epidemiology*

The disease is three times more common in women than in men. The peak age of onset is 30–50 years.

*Aetiology—specific issues*

This is unknown. A number of environmental agents have been implicated, for example, silica, industrial solvents.

*Clinical features*

Scleroderma (skin thickening) is the most characteristic clinical feature (Fig. 36). Raynaud's phenomenon is often severe. Look also for digital pitting (Fig. 37) (reflecting recurrent episodes of digital ischaemia), telangiectases, contractures (e.g. at the fingers, wrists, and elbows), basal crackles (a sign of lung fibrosis), and other signs of internal organ involvement. Dysphagia is common, resulting from oesophageal dysmotility.

*Investigations*

These are indicated to document internal organ involvement (e.g. chest X-ray, pulmonary function tests) (Fig. 38). Anticentromere antibodies are associated with limited cutaneous disease and anti-Scl-70 (antitopoisomerase) antibodies with diffuse cutaneous disease.

*Management*

Although there is no 'curative' treatment, therapies are available for the different organ-based manifestations (e.g. proton pump inhibitors for oesophageal reflux, vasodilators for Raynaud's phenomenon). Steroids are seldom used.

*Clinical course*

This is dependent upon the degree of internal organ involvement.

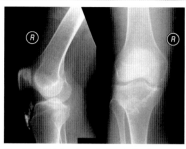

**Fig. 35** Calcinosis anterior to the knee in a patient with systemic sclerosis. Calcinosis most commonly occurs over pressure points.

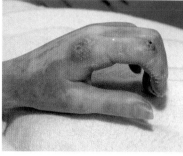

**Fig. 36** Marked skin thickening of the fingers and hand in a patient with diffuse cutaneous systemic sclerosis. Note the marked finger contractures and the areas of healed ulceration over the MCP and PIP joints of the index finger.

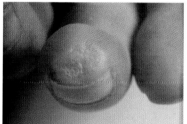

**Fig. 37** Digital pitting in systemic sclerosis.

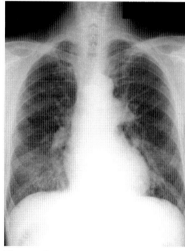

**Fig. 38** Basal fibrosis in systemic sclerosis.

# 13 Inflammatory muscle disease (polymyositis and dermatomyositis)

Inflammatory muscle disease is characterised by inflammation of striated muscle ('polymyositis'). If this occurs in association with inflammation of the skin it is termed 'dermatomyositis'. In older patients there is thought to be an association between dermatomyositis and malignancy.

*Epidemiology*

Female:male ratio is 2 to 3:1. There are two peak ages of onset—in childhood and in middle/late adulthood. This peak in childhood relates to dermatomyositis; polymyositis in the absence of skin involvement is rare in childhood.

*Clinical features*

The main clinical feature is proximal muscle weakness. The rash of dermatomyositis most commonly affects the face (sometimes with periorbital oedema, with heliotrope discoloration of the upper eyelids) and the extensor aspects of the hands (Fig. 39). Erythematous plaques over the dorsal aspects of the small joint of the hands are termed Gottron's papules. Subcutaneous calcinosis occurs in childhood dermatomyositis. Raynaud's phenomenon is common. Dysphagia and respiratory involvement are worrying features, suggesting progression of the disease to involve the pharynx and respiratory muscles.

*Investigations*

Muscle enzyme levels (including creatine phosphokinase) are usually high in active disease. Most patients demonstrate abnormalities on electromyography (EMG). MR scanning of muscles shows inflammation when the disease is active (Fig. 40). A normal muscle biopsy does not exclude the diagnosis as the disease is 'patchy'.

*Treatment*

This is with corticosteroids and/or immunosuppressants.

*Clinical course*

Some patients have a short self-limiting disease, while others have persistent disease with exacerbations and remissions.

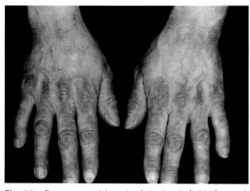

**Fig. 39** Dermatomyositis rash of the hands (with Gottron's papules).

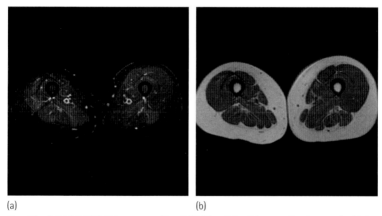

(a)                                  (b)

**Fig. 40** Axial (a) STIR (fat suppressed) and (b) T1 weighted images showing patchy high signal change due to muscle inflammation in the STIR image. Fat replacement (seen as high signal in the muscle on the T1 weighted image) can also be seen in these patients.

Sjögren's syndrome can be primary (occurring in the absence of other autoimmune diseases) or secondary (associated with other autoimmune diseases). It affects predominantly the exocrine glands, leading to decreased exocrine secretions.

*Epidemiology*

The female:male ratio is 9:1, with a peak age of onset of 30–50 years.

*Clinical features*

Sjögren's syndrome, when severe, can be extremely distressing. The main symptoms are dry, gritty eyes (kertatoconjunctivitis sicca) and a dry mouth (xerostomia), which can lead to difficulty swallowing dry food. Vaginal dryness also occurs. The parotid glands may be enlarged (Fig. 41). Other clinical features include Raynaud's phenomenon, arthralgia/arthritis, renal tubular acidosis, and interstitial lung disease. Sjögren's syndrome is associated with an increased risk of lymphoid malignancy.

*Investigations*

A high proportion of patients with Sjögren's syndrome have anti-Ro and/or anti-La antibodies. Reduced tear secretion can be detected by Schirmer's tear test (Fig. 42)—wetting of the filter paper by less than 5 mm per 5 minutes suggests impaired secretion. Other investigations include slit-lamp examination after Rose Bengal staining (this demonstrates keratiti); (Fig. 43) and minor salivary gland biopsy.

*Treatment*

This is often unsatisfactory. Artifical tears and saliva substitutes may be helpful. A key point is strict attention to dental hygiene, as patients are at risk of severe caries. Pilocarpine hydrochloride may be indicated for severe xerostomia.

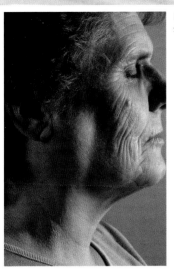

**Fig. 41** Parotid enlargement in Sjogren's syndrome.

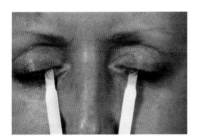

**Fig. 42** Schirmer's test showing wetting of the filter paper on both right and left.

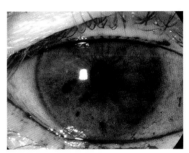

**Fig. 43** Rose Bengal staining in a patient with Sjogren's syndrome, demostrating uptake of the stain in the cornea. Courtesy of J. Kwartz.

The vasculitides are characterised by inflammation of blood vessel walls. Most are uncommon (exceptions are Henoch-Schönlein purpura in children and giant cell (temporal) arteritis in the elderly) and diagnosis may be difficult. Always suspect the diagnosis in an unwell patient with a multisystem inflammatory disease. Infarction and haemorrhage of internal organs are the most feared features of this group of diseases, which can be life-threatening. Classification of the vasculitides is usually based on the size of the blood vessel affected by the inflammatory process.

Vasculitis can also occur in association with other diseases, for example, rheumatoid arthritis and Sjögren's syndrome, emphasising how different immunologically mediated diseases overlap. Where possible, the diagnosis of vasculitis should be confirmed histologically.

## Wegener's granulomatosis

Small and medium blood vessels are involved. The peak age of onset is in the 40s. While the disease can involve all organs, key areas are upper respiratory tract (including sinusitis, nasal ulcers), the lungs (including pulmonary haemorrhage, pulmonary infiltrates), the eye (scleritis, proptosis (as a result of granulomatous inflammation causing an orbital mass; Fig. 44), and the kidney (glomerulonephritis). Constitutional symptoms (fever, weight loss), common to all the vasculitides, can be severe. Antibodies to the diffuse cytoplasmic form of antineutrophil cytoplasmic antibody (ANCA) are highly specific for Wegener's granulomatosis (Fig. 45).

## Polyarteritis nodosa

As with Wegener's granulomatosis, this affects small and medium sized vessels. Children can be affected. Polyarteritis nodosa can be associated with hepatitis B. Key clinical features include palpable purpura, digital ischaemia, abdominal pain (due to vasculitis), renal and neurological involvement.

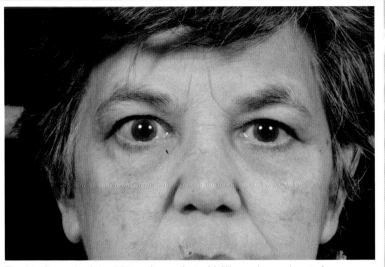

Fig. 44 Proptosis of the right eye in a patient with Wegener's granulomatosis.

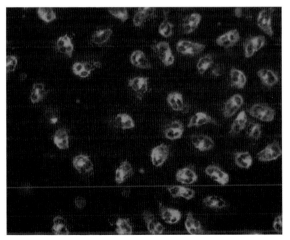

Fig. 45 Cytoplasmic ANCA—granular cytoplasmic staining with central interlobular accentuation. Courtesy of A. Moran.

## Churg–Strauss syndrome

Small and medium blood vessels are affected. Pulmonary manifestations are often prominent (and asthma usually precedes the systemic manifestations) and there may be eosinophilia.

## Behcet's syndrome

This disease of small and medium blood vessels is commonest in Japan and around the Mediterranean. Young adults are mainly affected. Key clinical features are recurrent oral and genital ulceration (Fig. 46), eye involvement (uveitis and retinal vasculitis), and vascular problems (thrombophlebitis, venous thrombosis).

## Small vessel vasculitis

This mainly affects the skin (Fig. 47) and occurs in association with a variety of disease processes, including drug hypersensitivity, infections, and Henoch–Schönlein purpura (predominantly a disease of children, characterised by nephritis, arthritis, and gastrointestinal manifestations as well as by a purpuric rash).

## Polymyalgia rheumatica and giant cell arteritis

Polymyalgia rheumatica is a disease of the elderly (it is rare below the age of 50 years), characterised by pain and stiffness of the shoulder and pelvic girdles and a high ESR. There is a dramatic response to moderate dose steroids.

There is an association between polymyalgia rheumatica and giant cell arteritis, which affects large arteries (sometimes termed 'cranial arteritis' because there is a high incidence of head and neck involvement, or 'temporal arteritis' because the temporal arteries are often involved). Clinical features of giant cell arteritis include headaches, scalp tenderness (around the temporal arteries), visual disturbances (including sudden blindness), and jaw claudication. It is a medical emergency: high dose steroids may prevent permanent blindness.

## Takayasu's arteritis

This is an uncommon disease of the aorta and its major branches. Young women (age less than 40 years) are mainly affected. Clinical features include headaches, visual disturbances, and limb claudication. The diagnostic test is arteriography.

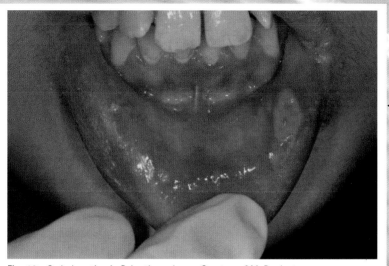

Fig. 46  Oral ulceration in Behcet's syndrome. Courtesy of M. Pemberton.

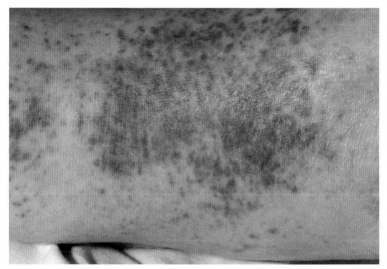

Fig. 47  Vasculitic rash.

# 16 Osteoarthritis

Osteoarthritis (OA) is the commonest joint disease and affects most people at some stage in their life. There are several typical patterns of osteoarthritis although not all patients fit into these.

*Epidemiology*

Osteoarthritis is extremely common and the prevalence increases markedly with age; 80% of older patients (>70) have symptomatic OA of at least one joint. All patients over the age of 60 prove to have osteoarthritis at autopsy. X-ray changes are present in over 50% of knees in patients over 65.

*Aetiology*

This condition involves degeneration and loss of articular cartilage, which is the bearing surface of synovial joints (Fig. 48). The pathology of the condition is now quite well characterised, and involves the production of degradative enzymes within the joint. The previous view that it is simply due to 'wear and tear' is no longer tenable. OA usually occurs in older patients ('idiopathic OA'), but it may occur secondary to joint deformity where excessive pressure on articular cartilage occurs (e.g. developmental dysplasia of the hip), or to joint injury (including sepsis), or to joint diseases such as gout (Figs 49 & 50). There is increasing recognition that osteoarthritis has a partial genetic component and tends to run in families.

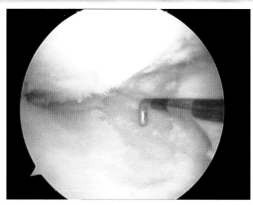

**Fig. 48** Osteoarthritis of the knee—there is severe fibrillation of the knee cartilage seen at arthroscopy.

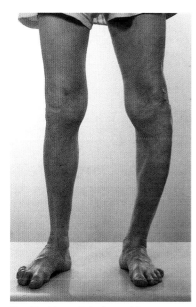

**Fig. 49** Varus of the knee—this predisposes to medial osteoarthritis. (Reproduced with permission from Andrew JG, Herrick AL, Marsh DR. Musculoskeletal Medicine and Surgery. Elsevier-Churchill Livingstone, Edinburgh, 2000.)

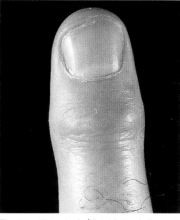

**Fig. 50** Heberden's (distal interphalangeal joint (IPJ)) and Bouchard's (proximal IPJ) nodes—these are due to osteophytes and are characteristic of small joint osteoarthritis. (Reproduced with permission from Andrew JG, Herrick AL, Marsh DR. Musculoskeletal Medicine and Surgery. Elsevier-Churchill Livingstone, Edinburgh, 2000.)

## Symptoms

Osteoarthritis may affect many small joints (this is especially common in middle-aged females), typically including fingers and small joints of the back (one cause of back pain). Another pattern is for it to affect one or more large joints, particularly in the lower limbs (hips, knees). Symptoms may be severe with limitation of movement, difficulty walking, and sleep disturbance. Stiffness and gelling may occur after rest or in the morning, although this is not as prolonged as in inflammatory joint disease such as rheumatoid arthritis. Joints that are asymptomatic despite the presence of osteoarthritis are frequent; symptoms may change from minimal to severe quite quickly in these joints (e.g. after trauma).

## Signs

There may be restricted range of movement in all planes. Pain and crepitus on movement are typical features. Osteophytes may be palpable (e.g. Heberden's nodes at the distal interphalangeal joints of the fingers) (see Fig. 50). An effusion may be present in the joint but this is variable; little or no synovial thickening is usually present (compare rheumatoid arthritis).

*Investigations*

Blood tests are normal. X-rays typically show joint space narrowing, small cysts (often multiple), osteophytes (small lumps of new bone formation at the periphery of the joint), and sclerosis of the subchondral bone (Figs 51–53). Deformity may be visible (e.g. a varus deformity at the knee, dysplasia of the hip). Because of the extremely common nature of osteoarthritis, the condition frequently coexists with other pathology (e.g. metastatic disease) and it is important not to attribute symptoms to osteoarthritis too readily.

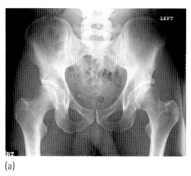

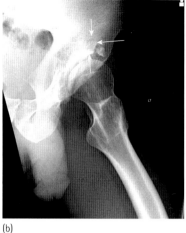

(a)  (b)

**Fig. 51**  Early osteoarthritis of the hip—there is hip dysplasia and an anterior cyst (arrowed on the lateral view).

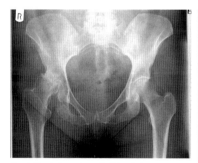

**Fig. 52**  Late osteoarthritis of the hip—there is complete loss of joint space and there are several cysts.

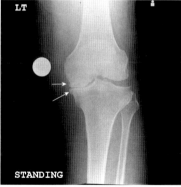

**Fig. 53**  Osteoarthritis of the knee—there are osteophytes (arrowed) medially and loss of medial joint space.

*Management*

The keystones of osteoarthritis management are pain relief, maintenance of mobility (including physiotherapy, weight loss, graded exercise) and use of walking aids. It is best to start treatment with simple analgesia (paracetamol and codeine). Some patients benefit from NSAIDs, but many do not and there are risks with these drugs. Some patients have a significant inflammatory component to osteoarthritis, but in most patients this is a noninflammatory condition. Thus, a few patients get an excellent result with injections into the joint of local anaesthetic and long-acting steroid, but most get only a brief period of relief and the value of such treatment is contentious.

Various surgical treatments may be offered including arthrodesis of joints (surgical stiffening of the joint) (Fig. 54) and osteotomy (realignment of the joint to ensure that pressure is spread equally across the joint; commonly done to treat early osteoarthritis of the knee by realigning a varus deformity of the tibia below the knee).

Total joint replacement is a good treatment for end-stage arthritis in many joints (Fig. 55). This usually gives dramatic relief of joint pain, but risks include joint sepsis, dislocation, and thromboembolism. The provision of total hip and knee replacement in particular has transformed the outlook for patients with end-stage disease of these joints. Very large numbers of such operations are now performed (>100 000 per annum in UK). The most common type of total joint replacements have one hard bearing surface (i.e. metal or ceramic) and one surface of ultrahigh-molecular-weight polyethylene (Fig. 56).

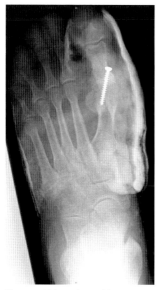

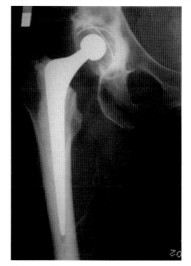

**Fig. 56** Picture of total hip replacement prosthesis.

**Fig. 54** This patient with osteoarthritis of the first metatarsophalangeal joint has undergone a fusion of the joint. There is a screw across the joint and a plaster cast supports the bones while they heal together.

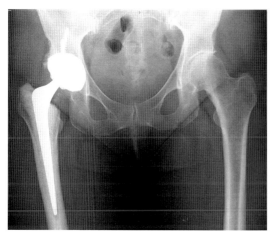

**Fig. 55** A right total hip replacement has been performed.

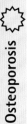
# 17  Osteoporosis

| | |
|---|---|
| *Definition* | Osteoporosis is characterised by loss and microarchitectural disruption of bone. It can be localised (for example, during disuse of a limb after fracture) or generalised. The World Health Organisation defines osteoporosis on the basis of bone mineral density—more than 2.5 standard deviations below the young adult mean. |
| *Epidemiology* | Osteoporosis is commonest in elderly women, but is a serious problem also in men. The incidence is increasing (reflected in the increasing incidence of hip fractures). |
| *Aetiology* | There is an uncoupling of the normally tight balance between bone resorption and bone formation. Risk factors for osteoporosis include increasing age, female sex (with loss of oestrogen post-menopausally), early menopause, race (white people are most affected), poor dietary calcium intake, smoking, corticosteroid use, immobility, and family history. |
| *Clinical features* | The clinical consequence of osteoporosis is fracture (often with minimal trauma). Common sites include thoracic and lumbar vertebrae (leading to back pain), proximal femur, distal radius (Fig. 57), and proximal humerus. Some patients present with progressive vertebral deformity with kyphosis (Fig. 58). |
| *Investigations* | The diagnosis of osteoporosis is usually made on bone densitometry. Plain radiographs are inaccurate, but demonstrate vertebral collapse in advanced disease (Fig. 59). Investigations such as FBC, ESR, biochemical screen, and myeloma screen help exclude underlying conditions (e.g. osteomalacia). |
| *Management* | This includes prevention (including screening of at risk groups) as well as treatment of established disease. Key points are: |

- Lifestyle measures (calcium intake, exercise, smoking cessation)
- Fall prevention
- Prophylactic treatment for patients on corticosteroids
- Drug treatment. Drugs include calcium and vitamin D, bisphosphonates, and selective oestrogen receptor modulators. Hormone replacement therapy is no longer a first-line approach

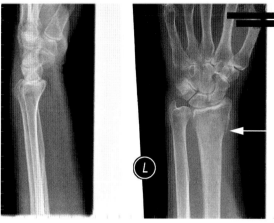

Fig 57   Fracture (arrow) of distal radius with minimal angulation.

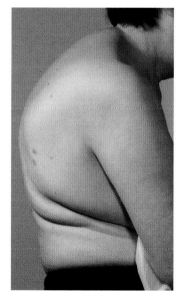

Fig. 58   Kyphosis (this patient was on steroids for vasculitis).

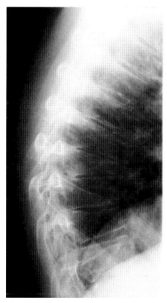

Fig. 59   Osteoporotic vertebral collapse, with anterior wedging. The anterior height of the vertebral body is more than 20% reduced compared to the posterior height.

# 18 Osteomalacia and rickets

*Definition* | In osteomalacia and rickets there is abnormal mineralisation of the skeleton (mature and growing, respectively).

*Epidemiology* | These are uncommon diseases in the West, but commoner in some ethnic groups, for example, Asian females.

*Aetiology* | Vitamin D deficiency leads to defective calcium absorption in the gut and decreased bone formation by osteoblasts (with the result that unmineralised osteoid is laid down). Predisposing factors for osteomalacia include renal disease, a diet poor in vitamin D, lack of sunlight exposure, malabsorption due to gut disease, and certain drugs (e.g. anticonvulsants).

*Clinical features* | Presenting features of osteomalacia include lethargy, aching pains, and muscle weakness. Some patients present with fracture. Childhood rickets leads to deformities during growth, including genu varum (bowing of the femur and tibia), bossing of the costochondral junctions ('rickety rosary'), and a transverse sulcus in the lower chest caused by the pull of the diaphragm on the softened ribs (Harrison's sulcus) (Fig. 60).

*Investigations* | Typically blood tests show a raised alkaline phosphatase, a marginally low calcium, and a low phosphate. Serum vitamin D should be assayed. The characteristic radiological feature of osteomalacia is the Looser's zone (pseudofracture) (Fig. 61). In rickets, the growth plate is widened and has a 'ragged' appearance.

*Management* | Treatment is with vitamin D replacement and calcium (with monitoring of calcium and phosphate concentrations). In renal osteomalacia, hydroxylated vitamin D (dihydrocalciferol) is required, to bypass the hydroxylation step in the kidney. In rickets, corrective osteotomies, especially around the knee, may be required for established deformity.

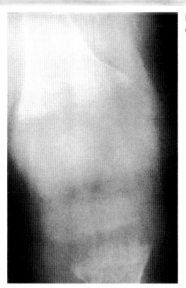

**Fig. 60** Widening and irregularity of the epiphyseal plate which is typical in rickets.

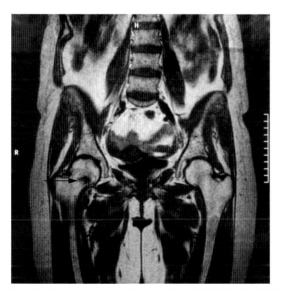

**Fig. 61** T1 weighted image in the coronal plane. There is a low signal line arising from the medial aspect of the right femoral neck. This is typical of a fracture. The incomplete nature of the fracture and its position would indicate a Looser's zone.

# 19 Hyperparathyroidism and hypercalcaemia

*Aetiology*

Excessive secretion of parathyroid hormone can be a primary endocrine disease (usually a single adenoma) or secondary to low serum calcium (e.g. in renal disease). Persistent overactivity of the parathyroid glands in chronic renal disease may lead to an adenoma in one of the glands (tertiary hyperparathyroidism). Parathyroid hormone increases serum calcium by increasing bone resorption and decreasing urinary excretion of calcium. Other causes of hypercalcaemia include bone malignancy (metastatic disease or multiple myeloma; Fig. 62) and rarer causes such as vitamin D intoxication, sarcoidosis, and thyrotoxicosis.

*Clinical features*

Hypercalcaemia causes muscle weakness, lethargy, polyuria and dehydration, mental changes including disorientation, and renal calculi. Primary hyperparathyroidism may present with these features of hypercalcaemia, with bone changes (see below) which result from the bone resorptive effects of parathyroid hormone, or with pseudogout. Secondary hyperparathyroidism in patients with renal disease is associated with osteomalacia.

*Investigations*

Blood calcium level is raised, and in primary hyperparathyroidism phosphate levels are low and parathyroid hormone levels high. Alkaline phosphatase may be raised. Renal function should be checked. Primary hyperparathyroidism leads to a fall in bone density (cortical bone is especially affected); therefore, bone mineral density should be checked. Plain radiographs may demonstrate bone erosion especially in the terminal phalanges (Fig. 63) and (in end-stage disease) multiple bone cysts ('osteitis fibrosis cystica').

*Management*

Mild hypercalcaemia does not require treatment. Severe hypercalcaemia should be treated with rehydration. Other measures such as a loop diuretic or a bisphosphonate may be indicated. Long-term treatment is directed towards the underlying cause, for example, parathyroidectomy or radiotherapy for metastatic bone disease.

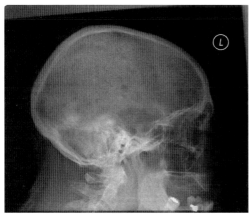

Fig. 62  Multiple lytic lesions in the diploic space of the skull vault typical of multiple myeloma.

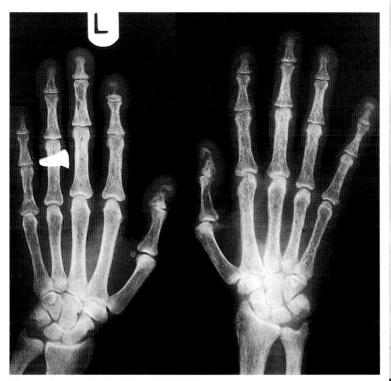

Fig. 63  Acro-osteolysis of the terminal phalanges.

# 20 Paget's disease (osteitis deformans)

This is a localised disease of bone remodelling (both bone formation and resorption are increased) resulting in disorganised architecture and a change in the mechanical properties of bone. Paget's can occur at single or at multiple sites.

*Epidemiology*

Paget's disease is common, usually presenting in older patients. It is particularly prevalent in the north of England.

*Clinical features*

Patients may present with bone pain and/or deformity. Common sites of involvement are the spine, the pelvis, the long bones (a characteristic finding being the 'sabre' tibia, with varus and procurvatum deformities; Fig. 64), and the skull (leading to frontal bossing and deafness due to compression of the auditory nerve in the petrous temporal bone). The brittle nature of pagetic bone means that patients are liable to fractures (fatigue fractures). Rarely osteosarcoma (highly malignant) may occur in an area of pagetic bone.

*Investigations*

An incidental finding of a raised alkaline phosphatase is often the presenting feature. The level of the alkaline phosphatase (and also of urinary hydroxyproline) is useful in monitoring disease activity and treatment response. Diagnosis is usually on the basis of the skeletal abnormalities on plain radiographs. The characteristic lesion is an expansile, sclerotic process (Figs 65a,b & 66). The differential diagnosis includes osteoblastic metastases (usually from prostate (see p. 54, see Fig. 68) or breast). Isotope bone scanning shows increased uptake at affected areas.

*Management*

Older patients with asymptomatic disease often do not require therapy. Bisphosphonates are the drugs most commonly used for symptomatic Paget's disease; calcitonin less frequently. Both inhibit osteoclast action and essentially slow down the abnormal bone remodelling.

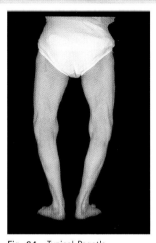

Fig. 64   Typical Paget's deformities of lower limbs.

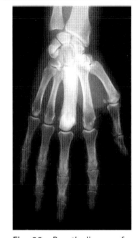

Fig. 66   Paget's disease of middle metacarpal. The bone is expanded and sclerotic. Paget's can affect any bone.

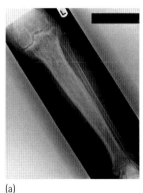

(a)

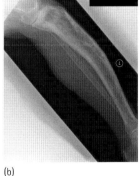

(b)

Fig. 65   (a) Anteroposterior and (b) lateral radiographs showing Paget's disease of tibia, with expanded, sclerotic bone (with a coarse trabecular pattern) and deformity. Note that the changes of Paget's disease commence at the end of a long bone and progress down the shaft.

## 21 Bone tumours

## Metastatic bone disease

Tumours metastasising to bone include carcinoma of the breast, lung, kidney, prostate, thyroid, and large bowel. Common sites are thoracic and lumbar spine, proximal femur, and proximal humerus.

*Clinical features*

The commonest symptom is pain, which is often unremitting and severe at night. Other presenting features may be pathological fractures or hypercalcaemia.

*Investigations*

The ESR and CRP are often high. Alkaline phosphatase is usually raised and sometimes the blood calcium. Prostate-specific antigen is raised in prostatic carcinoma. Plain radiographs may be normal in early disease but later will show lytic areas (Fig. 67) (or sclerotic lesions in prostatic or breast carcinoma; Fig. 68 ). Isotope bone scanning may show multiple lesions at a presymptomatic stage (Fig. 69). Multiple myeloma is associated with multiple lytic lesions (Fig. 70 and see Fig. 62), and if multiple myeloma is suspected, then serum protein electrophoresis (looking for a monoclonal band) should be checked and urine sent for Bence-Jones protein.

*Management*

Treatment of bone pain is palliative and includes radiotherapy. Surgery may be required to internally fix bones at risk of fracture, to stabilise the spine, or to decompress the spinal cord.

## Primary musculoskeletal tumours

These are rare; when they do occur this is usually in childhood and adolescence (see Fig. 101). Osteosarcoma is the commonest primary bone malignancy, usually occurring around the knee or in proximal humerus. Patients present with bone pain or a palpable mass. Sarcomata metastasise via the blood, leading to lung metastases. Plain radiographs show a variety of abnormalities including reactive new bone formation. MR determines the extent of the lesion. Definitive diagnosis requires biopsy, which should only be performed in specialist centres. Treatment has been revolutionised by multidrug chemotherapy.

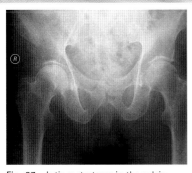

**Fig. 67** Lytic metastases in the pelvis above the right acetabulum. The cortical wall is destroyed (compare to the normal left side).

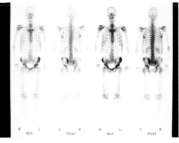

**Fig. 69** Multiple metastases of pelvis and L4. There is also some increased uptake of the shoulders and knees consistent with 'degenerative' joint disease.

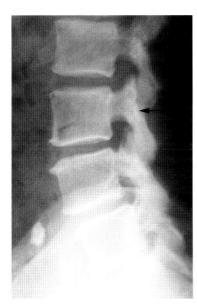

**Fig. 68** Diffuse sclerotic change affecting the posterior arch and spinous processes (arrow) in a patient with prostatic carcinoma. The lack of bone expansion indicates that appearances are those of metastases rather than those of Paget's disease.

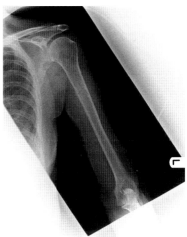

**Fig. 70** Multiple lytic lesions in the humeral diaphysis in a patient with multiple myeloma.

## 22 Bone infections (including tuberculosis)

| | |
|---|---|
| *Definition* | Osteomyelitis is infection of the bone or bone marrow. |
| *Aetiology* | A variety of organisms may cause osteomyelitis, including *Staphylococcus aureus* (including methicillin resistant, MRSA), *Pseudomonas* and *Mycobacterium tuberculosis*. Infection can arise by direct contamination (e.g. at a compound fracture, or after an operation) or by haematogenous spread. |
| *Clinical features* | There is usually pain and bony tenderness at the site of infection (Fig. 71). Adjacent joints may become swollen due to a 'sympathetic' effusion, although always consider the possibility that an adjacent joint may also be infected (septic arthritis). |
| *Investigations* | Plain radiographs will be normal in early disease. Later on, there will be bone rarefaction and periosteal new bone formation (Fig. 72). Bone sepsis will usually be associated with elevations in the ESR, CRP, and white blood count. While isotope bone scanning will detect a 'hot spot' in early osteomyelitis, appearances are nonspecific and MR imaging is now widely used (Fig. 73). White cell scans may also be useful. |
| *Management* | Early diagnosis is critical. Where at all possible, antibiotic therapy should be guided by isolation of the organism from tissue (obtained by biopsy) or pus. Protracted course of antibiotics required, usually 2 weeks of intravenous followed by 4 weeks of oral therapy. Surgery may be indicated to decompress bone or (if infection becomes chronic) to remove dead bone. |

## Tuberculosis of bones and joints

Although relatively rare, tuberculosis should always be considered in any atypical monoarthritis or bone or soft tissue tumour. The course of the disease is often slow and insidious. The spine may be affected (Fig. 74), leading to kyphosis. Skeletal tuberculosis requires a combined medical and surgical approach to management.

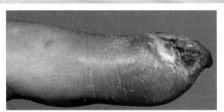

**Fig. 71** Osteomyelitis of the terminal phalanx of a patient with arterial insufficiency. Note the erythema and swelling proximal to the necrotic tissue.

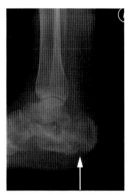

**Fig. 72** Osteomyelitis of the calcaneum with destruction of the cortex and of the subchondral bone inferiorly. There is a sequestrum (area of sclerotic dead bone; arrow).

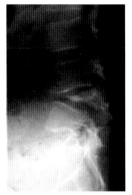

**Fig. 74** Spinal tuberculosis. There is a dense wedge-shaped gibbus (acute angulation of the spine)—a typical end-stage appearance of spinal tuberculosis.

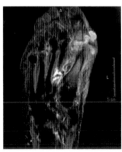

(a)

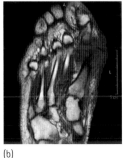

(b)

**Fig. 73** Septic arthritis and osteomyelitis of right great toe. (a) Fat-suppressed sequence showing affected marrow (high signal) compared to unaffected marrow (dark) in the other digits; (b) T1weighted sequence showing area of infection within the bone marrow as low signal (dark).

# 23 Medical conditions associated with musculoskeletal manifestations

Musculosketetal features occur in many diseases that are not primarily of the musculoskeletal system. Some important examples not included elsewhere are considered here.

## Erythema nodosum

*Definition*

This is an acute skin lesion caused by inflammation of subcutaneous fat, typically in young adults.

*Aetiology*

While many cases are idiopathic, a number of conditions are associated with erythema nodosum, including:

- Infection (e.g. streptococcal, tuberculosis)
- Drugs (e.g. sulphonamides, oral contraceptives)
- Sarcoidosis (see below)
- Lymphoma
- Inflammatory bowel disease

*Clinical features and treatment*

Tender nodules occur characteristically on the lower leg anteriorly (Fig. 75). There may be an acute arthropathy, which is self-limiting. Treatment is with rest and NSAIDs.

## Sarcoidosis

This is a systemic disease, characterised pathologically by noncaseating granulomata. It can be associated with either acute or chronic polyarthritis. The commonest articular presentation is with a self-limiting acute arthritis, often with erythema nodosum and hilar lymphadenopathy (Fig. 76). Large joints such as the ankles and knees are most commonly affected. Bone changes also occur, especially in chronic disease, typically affecting the digits with bone rarefaction, punched out ulcers, and bone destruction. Treatment of arthritis is with NSAIDs. Patients with active, persistent disease may require prednisolone.

## Dialysis arthropathy

Patients on long-term haemodialysis may develop a form of amyloidosis associated with high circulating levels of $\beta_2$-microglobulin. Chronic arthropathy (sometimes destructive) can develop. Carpal tunnel syndrome is a common feature.

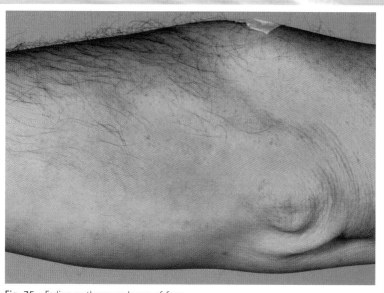

**Fig. 75** Fading erythema nodosum of forearm.

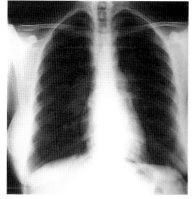

**Fig. 76** Hilar lymphadenopathy. (Reproduced with permission from Andrew JG, Herrick AL, Marsh DR. Musculoskeletal Medicine and Surgery. Elsevier-Churchill Livingstone, Edinburgh, 2000.)

# Neuropathic arthropathy

Patients with sensory neuropathy (most commonly diabetes) can develop an accelerated destructive joint disease ('Charcot's arthropathy'; Fig. 77). The affected joint(s) become(s) completely disorganised, with swelling and instability. Radiographs show gross destructive change, with bone resorption and new bone formation.

# Haematological diseases

*Haemophilia* Patients are at risk of intra-articular bleeding; the more severe the factor deficiency, the higher the risk. Presentation is with a monoarthritis, although with repeated episodes a more chronic arthropathy may develop.

*Sickle cell disease* Patients may experience a variety of musculoskeletal problems resulting from occlusion of blood vessels: painful crises (usually in the long bones), avascular necrosis, and dactylitis.

*Leukaemia* Patients, especially children, may present with joint pains and arthritis.

# Metabolic and endocrine disorders

*Haemochromatosis* Joint involvement typically affects the MCP joints of the index and middle fingers and may be the presenting feature of the disease. A proportion of patients present with calcium pyrophosphate dihydrate (CPPD) deposition disease.

*Diabetes mellitus* Associated musculoskeletal problems include diabetic cheiroarthropathy (a condition of the hands causing finger contractures and skin thickening), an increased risk of septic arthritis and osteomyelitis, neuropathic (Charcot) joints, forefoot problems (the 'diabetic foot'), resulting from microvascular and neuropathic changes, diffuse idiopathic skeletal hyperostosis (Fig. 78), and soft tissue problems including shoulder capsulitis and trigger finger.

*Thyroid disease* Proximal muscle weakness can occur with either hypo- or hyperthyroidism. Always check the thyroid function tests in the patient with generalised aches and pains.

# Malignancy

There are many associations between musculoskeletal disease and malignancy. Always suspect malignancy in the

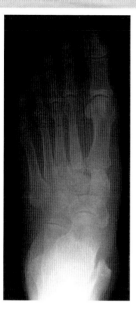

Fig. 77   A Charcot joint showing the destructive nature of the changes at the tarsometatarsal joints of the 1st and 2nd toes with multiple fragments. There is slight separation of the 1st and 2nd toes indicating ligamentous laxity.

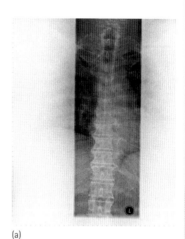

(a)

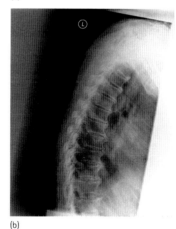

(b)

Fig. 78   (a) Anteroposterior view showing 'flowing' ankylosis of the lower thoracic spine. (b) The lateral view shows this continuing over at least 6 intervertebral disc spaces. For the diagnosis to be made a minimum of 3 consecutive disc spaces must be involved.

patient with musculoskeletal symptoms and suspicious features (e.g. weight loss, high ESR). Musculoskeletal symptoms may result from skeletal metastases (see Figs 67 & 69) or paraneoplastic syndromes (e.g. 'hypertrophic osteoarthropathy' in bronchial carcinoma).

# 24 Inflammatory joint disease in children

Chronic inflammatory arthritis in children (age at arthritis onset <16 years) is usually termed 'juvenile idiopathic arthritis'. It can be associated with major morbidity. Its classification is currently under review but three commonly recognised subtypes, defined by the pattern of disease in the first 6 months, are:

- Pauciarticular onset (arthritis occurs in 4 or fewer joints).
- Polyarticular onset (arthritis occurs in 5 or more joints). Some children (usually older girls) develop what is essentially rheumatoid arthritis.
- Systemic onset. Systemic features such as a high spiking fever and rash are prominent and may precede the arthritis.

*Epidemiology*

The prevalence has been estimated at around 1 in 1000 children.

*Aetiology*

This is unknown and is likely to be multifactorial.

*Clinical features*

Children may complain of surprisingly little pain. A parent may report how the child refuses to walk or crawl. Symptoms are often worst in the morning. On examination, children with 'Systemic onset' disease may have a high spiking fever, lymphadenopathy, and an evanescent, salmon-pink, macular rash (Fig. 79) (typically present during temperature spikes). Look for signs of joint inflammation (Fig. 80). The neck (Fig. 81) and temperomandibular joints are often affected. Particular points to highlight in children are:

- Contractures—these develop quickly, e.g. at knees and elbows
- Growth abnormalities

Generalised growth retardation occurs in systemic disease. Local growth abnormalities also occur, including:

- Overgrowth at the knee in the child with involvement of one knee (resulting in leg-length discrepancy and a compensatory scoliosis)
- Micrognathia due to mandibular hypoplasia

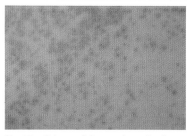

**Fig. 79** Salmon-pink, macular rash of juvenile idiopathic arthritis.

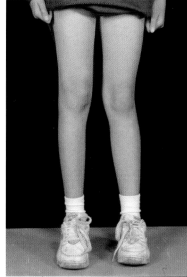

**Fig. 80** Right knee swelling in juvenile idiopathic arthritis—this girl had a limb length discrepancy.

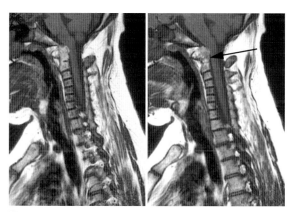

**Fig. 81** MR of neck in a patient with juvenile idiopathic arthritis. There is indentation of the anterior aspect of the cervical cord at C1. The marked picture shows erosive changes at C1/2 with erosion of the odontoid peg (arrow).

*Eye involvement*    A key point is that juvenile idiopathic arthritis can cause blindness through development of chronic anterior uveitis (Fig. 82). Young girls who are antinuclear antibody (ANA) positive are at particular risk. Most children are asymptomatic and therefore regular slit-lamp examination is required throughout childhood, to allow initiation of treatment at an early stage.

*Investigations*

ANA and rheumatoid factor should be checked. A positive rheumatoid factor is rarely found other than in those older children who go on to develop rheumatoid arthritis. There may be anaemia and a high ESR and CRP. Children with systemic onset disease often have high white blood count and platelet counts. Proteinuria may reflect amyloidosis, which occurs in a proportion of children with systemic onset disease. In some children, plain radiographs show erosions (Fig. 83).

*Differential diagnosis*

The main differential diagnosis is:

- Infectious/postinfectious, including rheumatic fever
- Other inflammatory diseases, e.g. SLE, vasculitis
- Malignancy, e.g. acute lymphoblastic leukaemia, neuroblastoma, bone tumour
- 'Structural', e.g. slipped femoral epiphysis
- Hypermobility (see p. 132)

*Management*

*Multidisciplinary team*    The principles of management are the same as those of adult polyarthritis. A multidisciplinary approach is essential, bearing in mind the particular needs of children; parents and school must be actively involved. Ophthalmologist, dietician, orthodontist/dentist, and child psychologist are all important members of the team. Many children benefit from hydrotherapy.

*Drug treatment*    Steroids are indicated in children with systemic disease unresponsive to NSAIDs. Methotrexate is the disease-modifying drug most commonly used. Increasing numbers of children are being prescribed biological agents including anti-TNF-$\alpha$ therapy.

*Surgery*    If joint replacement is indicated, then this should be performed in a specialist centre.

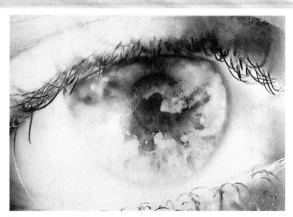

**Fig. 82**  Uveitis. (Reproduced with permission from Andrew JG, Herrick AL, Marsh DR. Musculoskeletal Medicine and Surgery. Elsevier-Churchill Livingstone, Edinburgh, 2000.)

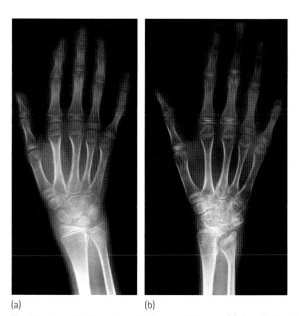

(a)  (b)

**Fig. 83**  Juvenile idiopathic arthritis—hand X-ray at (a) 'baseline' and (b) 18 months later showing marked erosive change of carpus and overall reduction in bone density. There is a secondary developmental deformity of the distal ulna.

# 25 — Shoulder problems

## Painful arc syndrome and rotator cuff tears

*Definition*

In painful arc syndrome, the arc of shoulder abduction is painful. The size of a rotator cuff tear may vary from minor to complete; supraspinatus is the most commonly affected muscle.

*Aetiology*

Several pathologies can cause a painful arc, most commonly supraspinatus tendonitis and subacromial bursitis (when the arc of abduction is painful between 60° and 120°). Subacromial bursitis can be associated with impingement (Fig. 84), commonly caused by an osteophyte at the tip of the acromium. Arthritis of the acromioclavicular joint causes a painful arc between 120° and 180°. Rotator cuff tears are a result of either trauma or degeneration due to age.

*Clinical features*

There is a painful arc. If the supraspinatus is torn, then initiation of abduction will be weak. The strength of the rotator cuff can be tested by examining resisted external rotation.

*Investigation*

Plain radiographs may demonstrate an osteophyte, calcification within the supraspinatus tendon or subacromial bursa (Fig. 85), or (in severe rotator cuff tear) loss of joint space (Fig. 86). Rotator cuff tears are demonstrated on ultrasound and MR scanning (Fig. 87).

*Management*

Painful arc is usually managed conservatively with physiotherapy, sometimes with local anaesthetic and steroid injection into the subacromial bursa. Impingement/cuff tears may require surgical decompression (usually arthroscopic). Cuff repair may also be indicated.

## Frozen shoulder (adhesive capsulitis)

This condition is of unknown aetiology and is most common in middle-aged females. Frozen shoulder gives rise to pain followed by severe stiffness with restricted movement. Treatment is with physiotherapy, intra-articular steroids, and occasionally manipulation under anaesthesia.

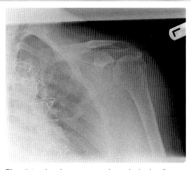

**Fig. 84** Impingement—there is lack of space between the greater tuberosity and the acromium, with some associated subchondral sclerosis.

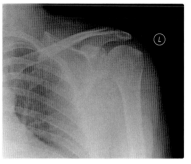

**Fig. 85** Calcification just above the greater tuberosity in the line of the supraspinatus tendon.

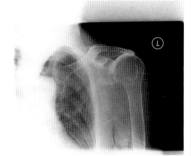

**Fig. 86** Subluxation of the humeral head and loss of joint space suggesting long-standing rotator cuff rupture.

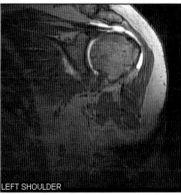

LEFT SHOULDER

**Fig. 87** Coronal oblique view of the shoulder (after injection of MR contrast). The fluid in the joint is high signal and can be seen in the joint and extending through the supraspinatus tendon and into the subacromial subdeltoid bursa. This is typical of a rotator cuff tear, which is full thickness.

## Enthesopathies: tennis elbow (lateral epicondylitis) and golfer's elbow (medial epicondylitis)

*Aetiology*

The pathological basis of these conditions is not well understood. Inflammation of the entheses (the anatomical structures where muscles arise from bone) often arises in patients without obvious overuse injury or systemic inflammatory disease.

*Clinical features*

In tennis elbow, pain is felt at the lateral epicondyle (often radiating distally) and is exacerbated by resisted wrist extension. In golfer's elbow, pain is felt at the medial epicondyle (again often radiating distally) and is exacerbated by resisted wrist flexion. Symptoms are usually worse with use of the forearm, for example, lifting weights.

*Investigations*

Blood tests are normal (unless there is an underlying systemic inflammatory disease) as are plain radiographs.

*Management*

Management options include physiotherapy, NSAIDs, an elbow splint (Fig. 88), and (if still no improvement) injection with local anaesthetic and steroid. Only rarely is surgical release required.

## Olecranon bursitis

This can occur on its own or in association with generalised conditions such as rheumatoid arthritis and gout. Pain is exacerbated by leaning on the elbow. If there is any suspicion of infection (Fig. 89), the bursa must be aspirated and the fluid sent for microscopy and culture. Occasionally persistent bursae require surgical removal.

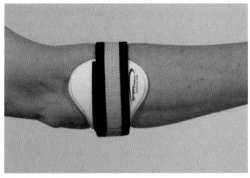

Fig. 88 Tennis elbow clasp.

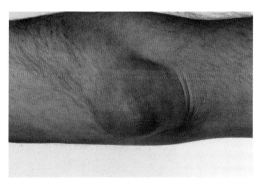

Fig. 89 Inflammed olecranon bursa—the concern is that this is infected.

# 27 Peripheral nerve problems affecting the distal upper limb

## Median nerve compression (carpal tunnel syndrome)

*Aetiology*

Most cases are idiopathic. Known causes include trauma (especially wrist fractures), pressure from hypertrophied synovium (e.g. in rheumatoid arthritis), diabetic mellitus, hypothyroidism, and pregnancy.

*Clinical features*

Pain and/or paraesthesia are felt in a median nerve distribution and are typically worst at night, often awaking the patient from sleep. On examination there may be sensory changes in a median nerve distribution, and in later stages there is wasting of the thenar muscles (Fig. 90). Symptoms may be provoked by tapping over the median nerve proximal to the transverse carpal ligament (Tinel's test) or by maintained wrist flexion (Phalen's test).

*Investigations*

Adequate diagnosis requires nerve conduction studies.

*Management*

This is usually surgical (decompression by division of the transverse carpal ligament, usually under local anaesthetic). Night splints and steroid injection into the carpal tunnel may be of benefit.

## Cubital tunnel syndrome/ulnar nerve dysfunction at the elbow

*Aetiology*

Most cases are idiopathic. Known causes include a cubitus valgus deformity and instability of the ulnar nerve.

*Clinical features*

Pain is felt at the medial side of the elbow, with radiation to the medial forearm and the ulnar 1½ fingers. Local pressure over the nerve may provoke symptoms. There may be signs of ulnar nerve motor dysfunction (intrinsic muscle weakness/ulnar claw hand—see below).

## Ulnar claw hand

This results from ulnar nerve dysfunction at elbow, forearm, or wrist. The deformity (hyperextension at the MCP joints of the ring and little finger, with flexion at the proximal and

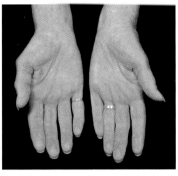

Fig. 90   Thenar wasting on right in a patient with carpal tunnel syndrome.

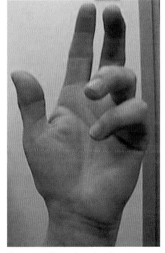

Fig. 91   Ulnar claw hand.

distal IP joints) results from weakness of the intrinsic muscles of the hand, almost all of which are supplied by the ulnar nerve (Fig. 91). The deformity is initially correctable but then becomes fixed (therefore physiotherapy and splintage are important aspects of management if recovery of nerve function is anticipated). If nerve compression is confirmed (by nerve conduction studies) then surgery should be considered.

## Ganglia

These are small cysts filled with viscous fluid (Fig. 92). They arise from outpouchings of the synovium, and are common around the wrist, where they can occur on either palmar or dorsal surface. If the ganglion is painful, and treatment is therefore required, then options are to aspirate with a wide-bore needle, to inject with steroid, or to excise. However, the ganglion may recur.

## Tenosynovitis

*Aetiology*

Inflammation of synovial tendon sheaths around the wrist occurs as a result of overuse and in inflammatory arthritis such as rheumatoid arthritis.

*Clinical features*

In rheumatoid arthritis, tenosynovitis most commonly affects the tendon sheaths on the dorsum of the wrist (Fig. 93). Tendon rupture can occur, leading to inability to extend at the MCP joints. A common form of tenosynovitis occurring in the absence of systemic inflammatory disease, and commonly associated with overuse, is de Quervain's stenosing tenosynovitis (involving abductor pollicis longus and extensor pollicis brevis). Pain is felt maximally around the radial styloid, associated with local tenderness and often swelling. Forced ulnar deviation of the wrist may cause severe pain (Finkelstein's test).

*Management*

Treatment is with NSAIDs and rest with wrist splintage. Injection of local anaesthetic and steroid may be indicated. Some patients require decompressive surgery.

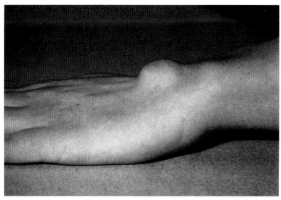

**Fig. 92** A dorsoradial wrist ganglion. (Reproduced with permission from Hooper, G. Orthopaedics (Colour Guide). Elsevier-Churchill Livingstone, Edinburgh, 1997.)

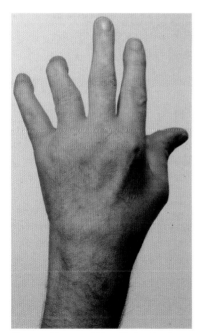

**Fig. 93** Rheumatoid hand/wrist showing extensor tendon sheath tenosynovitis. There is also a Z-thumb, and deformity of the ring and little fingers.

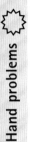

## Dupuytren's disease

*Epidemiology*

Males are more commonly affected, and at a younger age than women.

*Aetiology*

This fibrotic disease is most common in those with a family history of the disorder. There are associations with liver disease, diabetes, and anticonvulsants.

*Clinical features*

The ulnar side of the hand is most commonly affected. Patients initially report not being able to fully extend their fingers. On examination, initially there may only be a nodule of the palm or finger. As the disease progresses, there is fixed flexion deformity of one or more fingers, with contracture at the MCP and PIP joints (Fig. 94). Eventually very severe deformity may develop.

*Management*

The only effective management is surgery. The most commonly performed procedure is partial fasciectomy. Patients should be warned preoperatively about the risk of digital nerve injury, of incomplete correction, and/or possibility of recurrence.

## Trigger finger

'Triggering' of a finger (or thumb) is caused by a nodule developing in one of the flexor tendons and/or fibrosis and constriction of the finger flexor tendon sheath. The patient is aware of a flicking sensation on active flexion or extension of the digit. Trigger finger occurs especially in patients with rheumatoid arthritis or diabetes. Some trigger fingers settle spontaneously. Others require steroid injection into the tendon sheath or surgery.

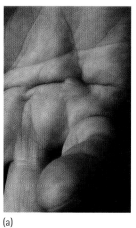
(a)

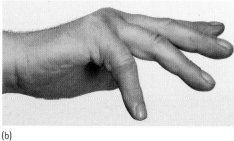
(b)

**Fig. 94** Dupuytren's contracture (a) in palm and (b) lateral view (the patient is attempting to extend his fingers).

**Lower limb disorders**

The lower limb is for standing and walking. Disorders of the lower limb affect these functions and limit mobility. Abnormal gait may be bilateral (e.g. festinant gait in Parkinson's disease) or unilateral (antalgic gait in osteoarthritic hip; usually visible as a limp).

## Hip disorders

The hip, due to its mechanics, experiences very high loads (up to six times body weight while running). Hip disorders are therefore common and frequently very painful.

*Clinical features*

### Symptoms

Patients usually experience pain from the hip as groin pain; it may radiate to the thigh, knee, or even the shin (Fig. 95). Pain at night is quite common. Stiffness in the hip results in difficulties in reaching the feet (and putting on socks and shoes).

### Signs

Patients may have a true leg length difference on inspection. There may be a fixed flexion deformity in the hip (Thomas's test). Hip movements are usually restricted relative to a normal hip (remember to compare the other side). Internal rotation is frequently the first range of movement to be reduced (particularly in osteoarthritis). Trendelenburg sign is often positive either due to mechanical inefficiency of the hip or to pain on single leg standing. Patients often limp.

*Investigations*

Plain X-rays of the pelvis and a lateral X-ray of the hip. Remember that this will irradiate the reproductive organs, so consideration is required about whether the investigation is needed. Remember that pain referred from the back can mimic many lower limb problems (Fig. 96). An MRI scan of the hip is particularly valuable in patients with avascular necrosis (which is often invisible initially on X-rays).

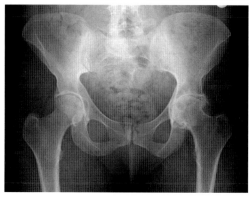

Fig. 95   This patient has osteoarthritis of the left hip with pain in groin and thigh.

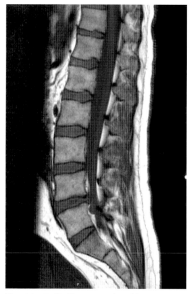

Fig. 96   L4/5 disc protrusion. Many symptoms in the lower limbs can arise in the spine—this patient also had cauda equina syndrome.

*Management*

Management of hip pain usually requires adequate analgesia (starting with simple analgesics); management of night pain may be particularly difficult. Use of a walking stick (typically in the opposite hand to the affected hip) is valuable. Surgery includes reduction of the hip (if dislocated in childhood or after trauma), osteotomy of the hip (to realign load transfer across the hip and make use of such articular cartilage as is still present), and total hip replacement (for end-stage disease).

## Avascular necrosis

This may occur in relatively young patients. Precipitating causes include steroid medication, excessive alcohol intake, Gaucher disease, and deep sea diving. Such patients frequently present with hip pain but normal X-rays and an MRI scan is often extremely helpful in diagnosis (Fig. 97).

## Trochanteric bursitis (inflammation of trochanteric bursa)

This is a very common condition of pain over the greater trochanter. Usually the hip joint itself is normal. Trochanteric bursitis is frequently associated with low back pain. Trochanteric bursitis is usually treated by injection of long-acting steroid and local anaesthetic.

## Paediatric hip disorders

There are four paediatric hip disorders of which you should be aware.

*Septic arthritis of the hip*    This may occur in all age groups of children, and is a serious emergency as it can cause high pressure within the hip joint causing complete destruction of the upper femoral epiphysis, with dire consequences for growth of the hip and subsequent permanent disability.

*Developmental dysplasia of the hip (DDH)* (Fig. 99)    This is commoner if there is a family history and in breech presentation babies. DDH varies from a mildly misshaped hip to complete dislocation of the hip. It is very important to detect this in the neonatal period, as the chances of a successful long-term outcome fall if treatment does not start until after the patient has started to walk. Treatment requires reduction of the dislocation and often further surgery as the anatomy of the acetabulum and femoral neck is abnormal even after the joint has been reduced. This condition is commoner in females.

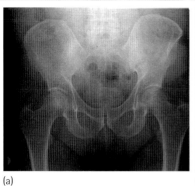 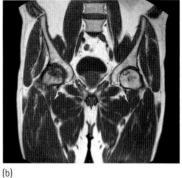

(a)                              (b)

**Fig. 97** This patient has avascular necrosis of both hips, more marked on the right. The plain X-ray appears normal, but a substantial area of avascular necrosis (AVN) is visible on the MRI scan. This is seen as a low signal area in the epiphysis, initially focal (a), but eventually extends to the articular surface. This is associated with articular collapse (b).

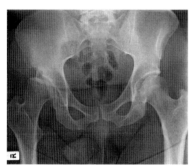

**Fig. 98** Evidence of right congenital dislocation of the hip in an adult.

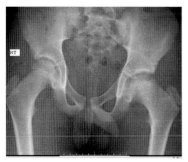

**Fig. 99** Perthes disease in a child (left hip).

*Perthes disease of the hip*    Perthes disease describes a misshapen hip due to repeated episodes of avascular necrosis (Fig. 99). Patients typically present at ages between 5 and 10 years. This is commoner in males. Treatment is controversial.

*Slipped capital femoral epiphysis*    Acute or chronic slip of the upper femoral epiphysis is a condition with presentation commonest between 10 and 15 years, especially in overweight male adolescents. The pain often radiates to the knee. Treatment is usually by fixation of the slipped epiphysis in situ. The condition is often bilateral (Fig. 100).

## Knee disorders

Beware of persistent knee pain in children and adolescents. The knee is the commonest site of primary bone tumours in these patients (Fig. 101).

*Clinical features*

### Symptoms

Knee problems are often marked by instability in the knee (giving way); this may be associated with 'pseudo locking' where the patient is unable to either flex or extend the knee due to pain. True locking indicates that the knee cannot be extended due to a mechanical block (e.g. torn meniscus or loose body). The site of pain in the knee is a good indicator of the likely pathology—pain at the front of the knee is usually due to patella pain (Fig. 102); pain at the joint line due to meniscal pathology (young patients) or osteoarthritis (older patients). Pain in the popliteal fossa on squatting is often due to posterior meniscal tears or arthritis.

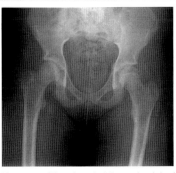
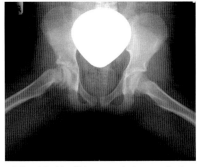

**Fig. 100** Slipped capital femoral epiphysis of the right hip. This may only be seen in the lateral view and it is essential to obtain both an AP and lateral view if this condition is suspected.

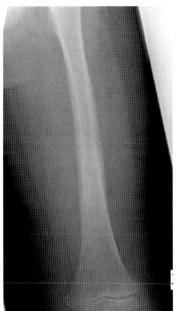
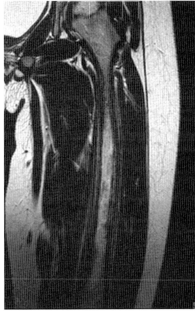

**Fig. 101** This child complained of knee pain. The plain film radiograph shows a periosteal reaction along the length of the shaft of the femur. There is loss of distinction of the cortical bone. The MR images shows signal change within the bone marrow and permiative changes of the cortex and pertiosteum inkeeping with an aggressive lesion. The diagnosis proved to be Ewing's sarcoma.

## Signs

Swellings around the knee may be due to bursae or Baker's cysts (in the popliteal fossa). Inspect for quadriceps wasting. An effusion in the knee joint is common. There may be malalignment of the knee (varus and valgus deformities are best seen on standing), and pain in the knee may be caused by local overloading of one part of the knee consequent on such deformities (thus varus in the knee often leads to medial tibiofemoral osteoarthritis). Tenderness in the affected area is usually present and may indicate the site of the problem. Patellofemoral crepitus is common on knee movement. Examine the knee ligaments and range of movement. Remember to ensure that the patient is able to straight leg raise (rupture of patella or quadriceps tendons may occur).

*Investigations*

Plain AP (standing) and lateral X-rays of the knee are very good at showing osteoarthritis and deformity. A skyline view is useful in patellofemoral problems. MRI scans are extremely useful to visualise meniscal tears and cruciate ligament injuries but are expensive and should be used appropriately.

*Management*

Analgesia is helpful. Physiotherapy and exercises are usually vital, especially in patellofemoral problems. Surgical treatment includes various arthroscopic manoeuvres including removal of torn menisci or of loose bodies and cruciate reconstruction. Partial or total knee replacements are effective treatment for end-stage disease (Fig. 103).

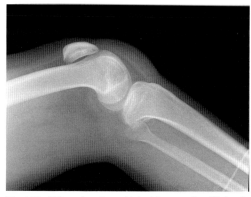

**Fig. 102** This patient has a high-riding patella—this is often associated with patella pain.

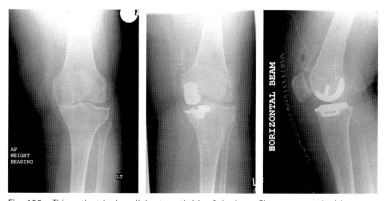

**Fig. 103** This patient had medial osteoarthritis of the knee. She was treated with a unicompartmental knee replacement.

# Foot disorders

These are common enough to support an entire profession (podiatry/chiropody). They are very common in older people, but serious foot problems also occur in inflammatory arthritis.

## Club foot (talipes)

This is a congenital disorder, sometimes associated with other developmental disorders (Fig. 104). Talipes calcaneo valgus is often self-correcting; talipes equino varus requires treatment (splinting) and often surgery.

## Hallux valgus

Valgus deformity is present at the first MTP joint, frequently associated with varus of the first metatarsal. Typically a painful exostosis develops on the neck of the metatarsal ('bunion'), which often rubs on shoes. This is treated with padding of footwear and supply of broad toe box shoes. Some patients need surgical correction of the deformity (Fig. 105).

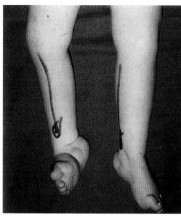

**Fig. 104** Congenital talipes equinovarus. (Reproduced with permission from Andrew JG, Herrick AL, Marsh DR. Musculoskeletal Medicine and Surgery. Elsevier-Churchill Livingstone, Edinburgh, 2000.)

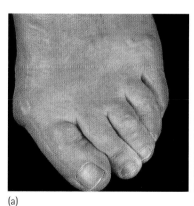

(a)

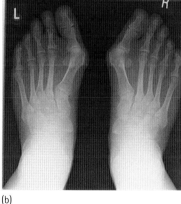

(b)

**Fig. 105** Hallux valgus. (Reproduced with permission from Andrew JG, Herrick AL, Marsh DR. Musculoskeletal Medicine and Surgery. Elsevier-Churchill Livingstone, Edinburgh, 2000.)

## Hallux rigidus

Hallux rigidus is osteoarthritis of the first MTP joint (Fig. 106). This is surprisingly common in young men. It is often treated with surgical fusion (arthrodesis).

## Hammer and claw toes

These typically occur in the second, third, and fourth toes. Hammer toe is hyperflexion at the proximal interphalangeal joint, with prominence of the PIP joint (where a painful callosity develops) and 'hammering' of the tip of the toe on the floor. Claw toes have excessive flexion at PIP and DIP joints; this is sometimes associated with neurological abnormality (spastic disorders). Surgical straightening may be required.

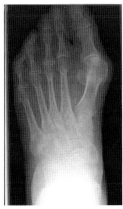

Fig. 106  Hallux rigidus—osteoarthritis of the first MTP joint.

'Mechanical' problems of the lumbar and cervical spine

*Definition*

'Mechanical' back or neck pain means that the pain is due either to overuse of a normal anatomical structure ('strain'), or to deformity or trauma of an anatomical structure. Mechanical back and neck pain are very common.

*Aetiology*

The main causes are:

- Trauma (includes 'whiplash injury')
- 'Degenerative' disease
  - Spondylosis (with loss of disc space and osteoarthritis of the apophyseal joints) (Fig. 107)
  - Disc herniation (Fig. 108)
  - Spondylolisthesis. Here there is forward displacement of a vertebrae relative to the one below. While this may be degenerative, other possible causes are congenital or traumatic (Fig. 109)
  - Spinal stenosis. Here there is narrowing of the spinal canal. While this may be degenerative (with disc bulge/prolapse or spondylolisthesis) it may also be congenital (or a combination of both)
- Post surgical back pain
- None of the above (sometimes termed 'muscle strain' or 'ligamentous strain').

Occupational factors are often important.

*Clinical features*

## Symptoms

Mechanical pain is usually worse on movement, or after standing or sitting. A sudden onset may indicate an acute disc prolapse. A detailed history is essential to (a) explore the possibility of another cause for spinal pain, e.g. infection or malignancy, and (b) determine whether there might be any neurological compromise, either lower motor

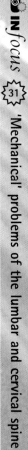

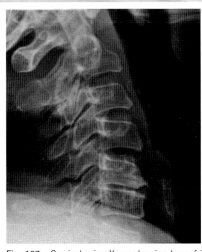

**Fig. 107** Cervical spine X-ray showing loss of joint space and osteophytes at C6/7 and facet joint disease.

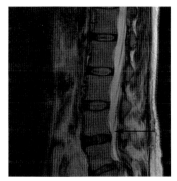

**Fig. 108** MR image (T2 weighted) showing loss of disc height, reduced disc signal, and bulging of the disc material into the anterior theca causing deviation of the transiting nerve root (arrow).

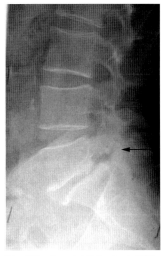

**Fig. 109** Spondylolisthesis at L5/S1. There is an anterior slip of L5 on S1, and a defect in the pars interarticularis of L5 (arrow).

neurone (radiculopathy at the level of the exiting nerve root) or upper motor neurone (spinal cord or cauda equina compression). Radicular pain is felt in the distribution of the affected nerve, and is usually caused by either a disc herniation or by osteophytes causing intervertebral canal stenosis (there may be a combination of both).

## Signs

A full examination is essential, looking for pointers to an unsuspected cause for spinal pain. Spinal movement may be limited and/or painful asymmetrically, depending upon the nature of the problem. Because spinal cord or nerve roots may be compromised, a full neurological examination is essential. Remember to perform the straight leg raising and femoral stretch tests (stretching the sciatic and femoral nerves, respectively). Positive tests indicate nerve root irritation.

*Investigations*

No investigations are necessary if the history is only short and the patient is otherwise well. If pain persists, or there is evidence of neurological compromise, then further investigation is required. In mechanical spinal pain, there is often a poor correlation between the severity of symptoms and the degree of 'degenerative' change on plain radiographs, which show loss of disc space, osteophytes, and osteoarthritis of the apophyseal (or 'facet') joints (Fig. 110; see Fig. 107). Flexion and extension views should be requested if spinal instability is suspected. CT scanning gives excellent demonstration of bone, for example in spinal stenosis, but does not demonstrate intradural lesions. MR scanning is usually the preferred imaging modality for the spine, allowing visualisation of intradural structures (see Fig. 108; Fig. 111).

*Management*

Many patients with mechanical spinal pain can be managed conservatively with patient education, analgesics, and physiotherapy. A minority will require surgery. The three main indications for surgery are:

1. Nerve root irritation (the radicular pain should be worse than the neck or back pain). This is the commonest indication for spinal surgery.
2. Spinal cord compression. Acute onset of spinal cord compression or cauda equina syndrome is a surgical emergency.
3. Instability (spinal fusion may be indicated).

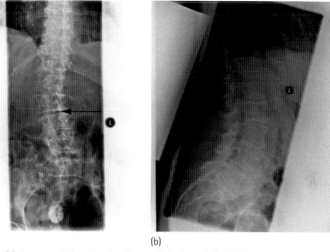

(a)                              (b)

**Fig. 110**   (a) Anteroposterior view showing scoliosis, loss of disc height, and marginal osteophytes. There is an area of low attenuation of the L3/4 disc space (arrows)—this is seen in 'degenerative' change. (b) Lateral view, showing loss of disc height and some loss of alignment with multiple small anterior osteophytes.

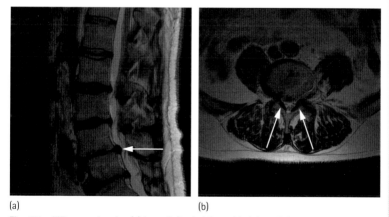

(a)                              (b)

**Fig. 111**   MR scans showing (a) loss of disc height and bulging of the disc into the anterior theca (arrow). The transverse image (b) shows degenerative change of the facet joints with associated thickening of the ligamentum flavum (arrows) which, combined with the central disc herniation, lead to spinal stenosis.

# 32 Nonmechanical causes of spinal pain

Nonmechanical causes of spinal pain

Low back and neck pain are common, and the vast majority of patients have 'mechanical' pain as described in the previous sections. However, other causes that require specific treatment should always be considered. They include the following.

*Inflammatory (noninfectious)*

These causes are described in the spondyloarthropathy sections (see pages 18, 20 & 24). Suspect spondyloarthropathy if the patient is stiff in the morning and the back pain relieved on exercise.

*Malignancy*

Metastatic disease or multiple myeloma are the most common causes of malignancy-associated back pain (see page 54). Suspect this if the pain is unremitting, bad at night, and there are worrying features such as weight loss.

*Infection*

Infective causes include vertebral osteomyelitis (see page 56), paravertebral abscess, and discitis (infection of the intervertebral disc, which can occur in isolation or in association with osteomyelitis) (Fig. 112). Suspect this if there are features of infection, for example fever, or a raised white blood count.

*Bone disorders*

These include osteoporotic vertebral collapse and Paget's disease (see pages 46 & 52).

*Nonspinal causes*

Spinal pain may be referred from elsewhere. For example, back pain may be referred from the hip or from the viscera (e.g. colonic or ovarian carcinoma, or abdominal aneurysm) and neck pain from the shoulder, from the viscera (e.g. oesophageal spasm), or from the diaphragm (e.g. subphrenic abscess).

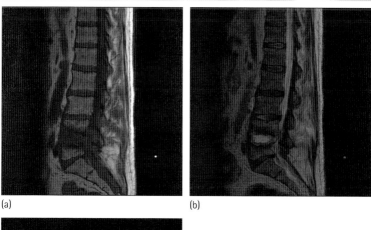

(a)  (b)

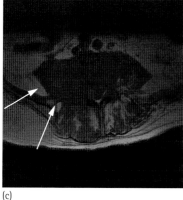

(c)

**Fig. 112**  Discitis. (a) T1 weighted MR image showing widening of the L4/5 disc space with destruction of the adjacent endplates with sclerosis and oedema. (b) T2 weighted MR image. The disc space widening can be seen to be a fluid collection (high signal). (c) T2 weighted transverse MR image. This shows some destruction of the right side of the vertebral body and extension of the inflammatory change into the paraspinal space (arrow). There is some compression of the nerve roots within the cord.

# 33 Multiple injuries

Patients with multiple injuries require systematic but decisive assessment and management, which are carried out simultaneously (Fig. 113). The use of the methods taught in advanced trauma life support courses has improved the outlook for these patients where it is easy to get management wrong.

*Epidemiology*

Multiple injuries mostly occur in young adults, but may affect any age. Worldwide, for patients aged 5 to 45 years trauma is second only to HIV/AIDS as a cause of death (about 3 million per year worldwide).

*Aetiology*

Road traffic accidents and falls predominate in the UK. Penetrating injuries (e.g. gunshot wounds) are common elsewhere.

*Management*

Airway, breathing, and circulation are always managed first. All patients should have supplemental oxygen provided and adequate intravenous access ensured. It is important to protect the cervical spine. An initial **primary survey** of airway, breathing, circulation, disability (neurological injury) and exposure is carried out. X-rays of chest, pelvis, and cervical spine are obtained. Bloods should be taken for cross match and base line measurement of FBC and U&Es.

After the primary survey is complete and the initial findings have been appropriately managed, a complete head to toe **secondary survey** is carried out. This includes assessment of all the body systems. While this is carried out it is important to pay close attention to the elements of the primary survey as these patients can deteriorate quickly from previously unrecognised injuries.

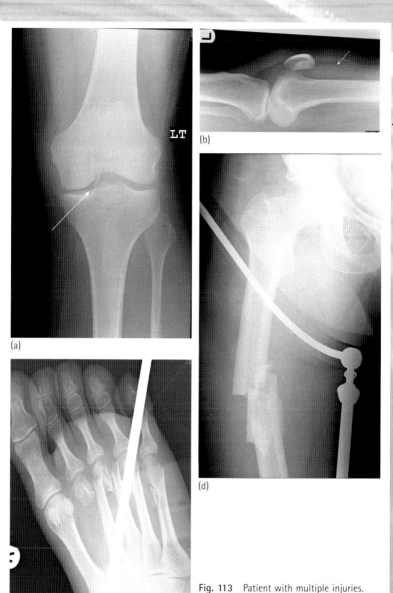

(a)

(b)

(d)

(c)

**Fig. 113** Patient with multiple injuries. The patient has a fracture in the left knee (a) causing a lipohaemarthrosis and fluid level (both arrowed) (b), multiple metatarsal fractures (c); and a fracture of the right femur (d).

# 34 Fracture atlas: upper limb fractures

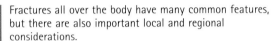

Fractures all over the body have many common features, but there are also important local and regional considerations.

*5th metacarpal neck fracture* (Fig. 114)   These are usually due to fighting! They generally require no treatment other than analgesia and support with a bandage. It is important to check that the fingers are not malrotated (inspect that the fingernails are correctly aligned when inspected end on).

*Scaphoid fracture*   This is the commonest carpal bone to be broken and is usually caused by a fall to the outstretched hand (Fig. 115). The fracture causes pain and tenderness in the anatomical snuff box at the base of the thumb. Fractures are sometimes invisible on the initial X-rays and hence are misdiagnosed as a wrist sprain. There is a risk of nonunion of the fracture (particularly if displaced); this eventually leads to wrist arthritis. If it is not possible to identify a fracture on X-ray but clinical suspicion is high, an MRI scan will reveal whether a fracture is present.

*Distal radius fracture*   This is common in all age groups. Children often suffer greenstick or buckle fractures (incomplete fractures) (Fig. 116). Adults may suffer Colles type fracture (dorsal angulation) or Smith's type fracture (palmar angulation). Both types of fracture may be simple (i.e. only two pieces) or very comminuted (i.e. many pieces). Acute median nerve compression (carpal tunnel syndrome) may occur and may need acute carpal tunnel release. The fracture is treated by reduction of the fracture and (in adults) increasingly frequently by wire or plate fixation.

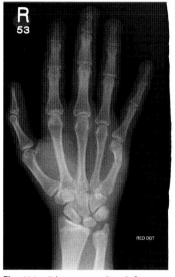

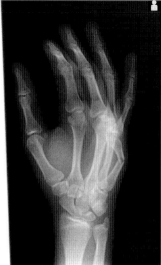

Fig. 114   5th metacarpal neck fracture.

Fig. 115   Scaphoid fracture.

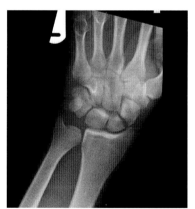

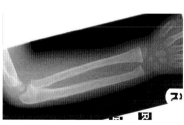

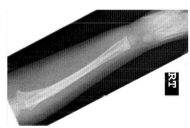

Fig. 116   Distal radial greenstick fracture in a child.

*Radial head/shaft fractures*   Both fracture types occur due to falls. Radial and ulna shaft fractures have the risk of impeding forearm rotation, so accurate reduction is essential. They are usually treated by a plate fixation in adults and accurate manipulation and plaster fixation in children. Radial head fractures (Fig. 117) affect elbow function but are frequently undisplaced and then only require early movement and physiotherapy.

*Supracondylar fracture of humerus*   These fractures are common in children; they may be associated with severe swelling and brachial artery damage, which can cause necrosis of forearm muscles (Volkmann's ischaemia). This leads to disastrous hand deformity and stiffness, so reduction of the fracture must be associated with careful assessment of the vascular tree (Fig. 118).

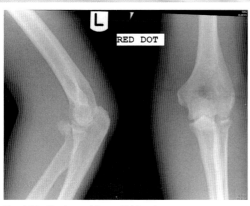

**Fig. 117** Fracture of the radial head.

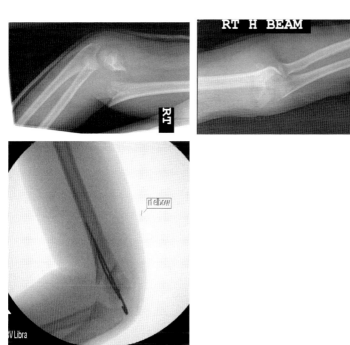

**Fig. 118** A displaced supracondylar fracture before and after fixation.

*Humeral shaft fractures* The radial nerve is vulnerable as it spirals around the humeral shaft. Injuries in this area may cause a radial nerve palsy and wrist drop. Fractures are often treated by conservative treatment (hanging cast or brace) or plate fixation (Fig. 119).

*Humeral neck fractures* This is a very common osteoporotic fracture, but also occurs in children (where a remarkable degree of remodelling of displaced fractures occurs) (Fig. 120). In older patients it usually results in some degree of permanent stiffness. The best treatment for these fractures is still very uncertain.

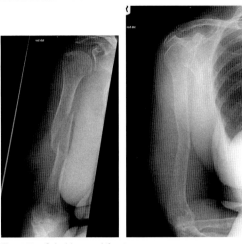

Fig. 119   Spiral humeral fracture.

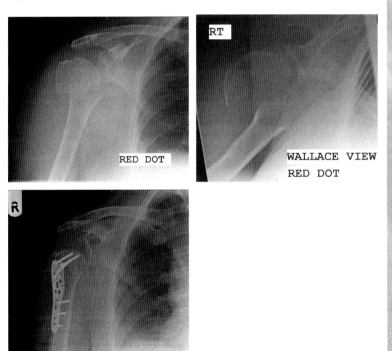

RT

RED DOT

WALLACE VIEW
RED DOT

Fig. 120   Fracture of neck of humerus before and after internal fixation.

Cervical spine fractures are alarming injuries due to the potential for disastrous spinal cord damage. Accordingly all neck injuries must be treated with care.

*Aetiology*

Cervical spine injuries are usually the result of high-energy accidents or falls; they also may occur as a result of evidently low-energy injuries in people with pre-existing neck problems (severe cervical spondylosis; ankylosing spondylitis).

*Clinical features*

### Symptoms

Neck pain and stiffness are usually present. The patient may complain of weakness, paraesthesiae, or difficulty passing urine.

### Signs

If you are suspicious of cervical spine injury, keep the neck immobilised until adequate investigations have been obtained. Tenderness in the neck and restriction of active movement may be present. There may be bruising (remember to look in the oropharynx for bruising due to an odontoid peg fracture) (Fig. 121). Weakness and decreased tone or change in sensation in the upper or lower limbs should be sought. Reflexes are usually diminished initially in both upper and lower motor neurone injuries. Spasticity and increased reflexes occur later.

*Investigations*

X-rays of the neck including a lateral view showing the upper border of T1 (C7/T1 junction is a frequent site of injury) and a through mouth odontoid peg view. A CT scan may be required simply to rule out an injury and is almost always obtained if a fracture is visible on the initial cervical spine X-ray.

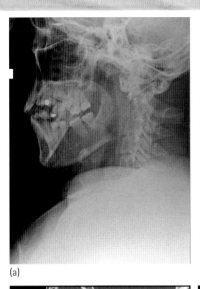

(a)

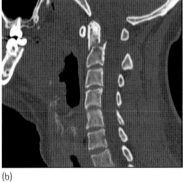

(b)

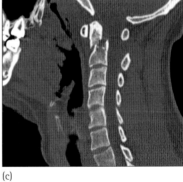

(c)

Fig. 121   Fracture of odontoid peg of C2—difficult to see on plain X-ray (a) but visible on spiral CT scan with sagittal reconstructions (a and b).

# Management of spinal injuries (cervical, thoracic, and lumbar)

Careful immobilisation is essential to prevent movement of the neck causing further damage (head blocks, patient nursed flat in bed). Consider referral to specialist spinal orthopaedic surgeon for assessment for surgical treatment. If there is neurological injury, refer the patient to a specialist spinal injuries unit. There is a severe risk of pressure area and bladder problems, blood pressure instability, and of other injuries being missed so careful and repeated examination is essential.

# Lumbar (and thoracic) spine fractures

Lumbar fractures may occur due to very low-energy injuries (extremely common in osteoporosis (Fig. 122)) or high-energy injuries (Fig. 123). The two require a radically different approach. Low-energy fractures in osteoporosis require a short period of rest and analgesia and then mobilisation and possibly physiotherapy. It is important to manage the osteoporosis.

High-energy lumbar or thoracic fractures (like cervical spine injuries) have a risk of injury to the spinal cord or cauda equina. Clinical assessment principles are similar to cervical spine fractures. Patients should be nursed flat in bed with log rolling when moving the patient. Surgical stabilisation is sometimes required and may permit more rapid mobilisation than the prolonged bed rest that is needed with conservative treatment.

# Pelvic fractures

These vary from minor low-energy fractures in osteoporotic patients (e.g. pubic ramus fracture) to severe high-energy fractures. High-energy fractures of the pelvis have the capacity for dramatic blood loss and should not be underestimated.

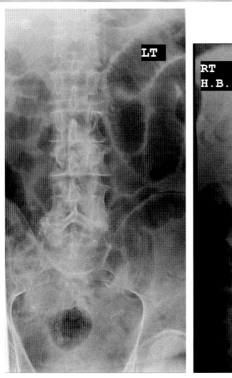
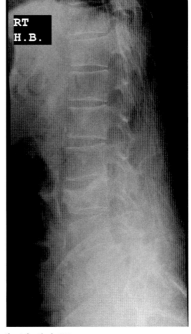

**Fig. 122** Osteoporotic fracture of L3 in a patient in their 80s.

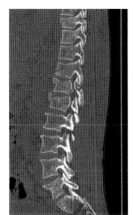
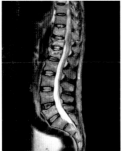
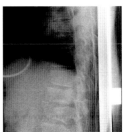

**Fig. 123** Fracture of T12 and L1 due to fall from a height in a young patient.

# 36 Fracture atlas: lower limb fractures

## Femoral neck fractures

Femoral neck fractures are the archetypal osteoporotic fracture; this is a serious injury in older patients with a high mortality rate (30% at 6 months).

*Epidemiology*

50 000 cases per year in the UK.

*Aetiology*

These fractures generally require a combination of osteoporosis and a fall. Prevention of both of these is the optimal method of reducing the burden of these fractures.

*Clinical features*

### Symptoms

The patient complains of severe pain at the hip and is usually (but not always) unable to walk.

### Signs

There is often shortening and externally rotation of the leg. There is pain on attempted hip movement. Patients with an undisplaced fracture (and no deformity) are usually unable to weight bear.

*Investigations*

Anteroposterior pelvis and lateral X-ray of the affected hip. Hip fractures may be extracapsular (typically intertrochanteric) or intracapsular (typically transcervical). Preoperative blood tests and other investigations are important to assess the patient's readiness for surgery.

*Management*

Almost all femoral neck fractures require operation. Extracapsular fractures are typically treated with a sliding screw and plate ('dynamic hip screw') (Fig. 124). Intracapsular fractures if displaced have a significant risk of avascular necrosis or nonunion of the femoral head, and are treated with a partial hip replacement (hemiarthroplasty) in older patients (Fig. 125). Undisplaced intracapsular fractures

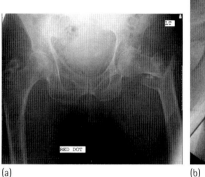
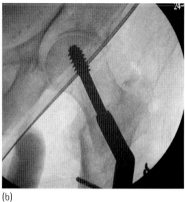

(a)  (b)

**Fig. 124** X-rays before (a) and after (b) internal fixation of an extracapsular intertrochanteric fracture of the femoral neck.

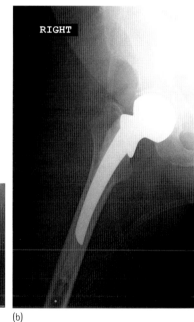
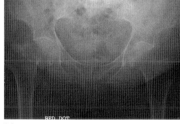

(a)  (b)

**Fig. 125** X-rays before (a) and after (b) hemiarthroplasty for an intracapsular fracture of the femoral neck.

in old patients and all intracapsular fractures in young patients are treated with screw fixation.

## Femoral shaft fractures

Femoral shaft fractures occur in all age groups. Substantial blood loss may occur. Children's fractures are usually treated with traction, although this approach is changing at present and internal fixation is more frequently used than it was. Adult fractures are usually treated with an intramedullary nail (a rod that permits screws to pass through the top and bottom part of the nail to prevent rotation or shortening of the bone; Fig. 126).

## Tibial plateau fractures

This is a common type of intra-articular fracture, usually due to falls. It is usually associated with a lipohaemarthrosis (marrow fat leaks into the knee, and can be seen in the aspirate together with the blood if the knee is aspirated). Damage to the articular surface may lead to later arthritis. Conservative treatment is possible, but most fractures are treated by internal fixation (Fig. 127). It is most important to achieve accurate reduction of the joint surface and then to permit joint movement to minimise stiffness and to protect the articular cartilage. The combination of accurate fixation of the joint surface and then early movement is usually the objective in intra-articular fractures.

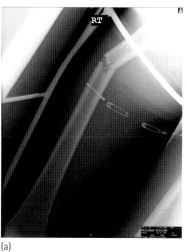
(a)

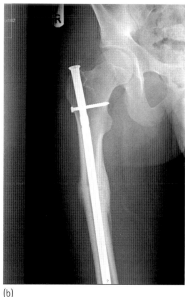
(b)

Fig. 126  Femoral shaft fracture before (a) and after (b) an intramedullary nail. There are also screws through the distal part of the nail to prevent malrotation of the femur.

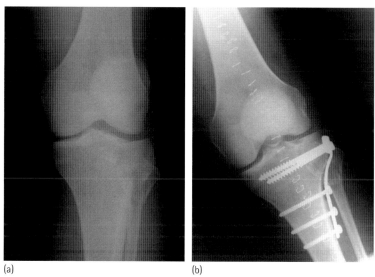
(a)                                    (b)

Fig. 127  Depressed lateral tibial plateau fracture before (a) and after (b) fixation.

# Tibial shaft fractures

This is a common injury in young adults, frequently occurring during football. It may be a transverse fracture (due to a bending force, such as being kicked on the shin) or a spiral fracture (due to a twisting force, such as falling with the foot fixed). Blood supply to this bone is relatively poor and fracture healing is sometimes slow. Even a normally healing fracture will require between 4 and 6 months before an adult is able to return to a job requiring mobility. Delayed union or nonunion are quite common, as are prolonged periods of disability due to the injury. Treatment may be with plaster, intramedullary nail, or external fixator (Figs 128 and 129). Open tibial fractures are common and meticulous care is required in the early management of such injuries to prevent subsequent bone infection, which is extremely difficult to eradicate.

Tibial shaft fractures are the commonest cause of compartment syndrome, but this may occur after most types of fracture. This describes the situation where, due to bleeding and swelling, the pressure within a muscular compartment rises above the capillary perfusion pressure. This results in marked ischaemia of the muscles and severe pain, with loss of active movement. The distal pulses are normal. Surgical decompression of the affected compartments is a surgical emergency.

# Ankle fractures

These are very common. Undisplaced fractures are treated conservatively in plaster. Displaced fractures (Fig. 130) are treated by internal fixation due to the risk of late

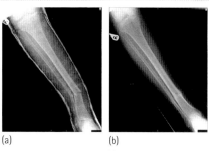

(a)     (b)

**Fig. 128** Patient before (a) and after (b) treatment for a tibial fracture. The fracture has healed with a small external callus. Only anteroposterior views are shown.

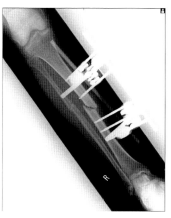

**Fig. 129** Tibial fracture with an external fixator applied.

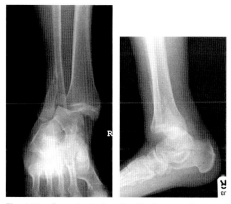

**Fig. 130** Severely displaced ankle fracture, fracture dislocation.

osteoarthritis if a good position of the joint surfaces is not maintained (Fig. 131).

## Foot fractures

These are common. They include calcaneal fractures (due to a fall from a height—they may be associated with other injuries especially lumbar fractures) (Fig. 132) and various forefoot fractures. Persistent pain for months is common as the foot is a heavily loaded structure.

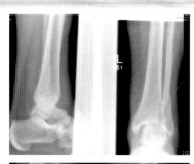

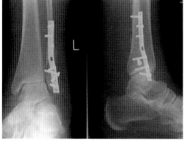

Fig. 131　Lateral malleolus fracture (arrow) with medial diastasis. Same fracture seen after fixation.

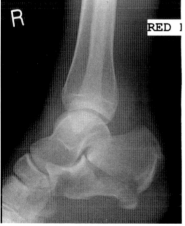

Fig. 132　Calcaneal fracture after a fall from a height.

# 37 Fracture atlas: fractures in the elderly

Fractures in elderly patients are increasingly common. Fracture management is difficult due to medical comorbidities, poor bone (bone fixation often weak), and the need for the patient to weight bear (weak muscles prevent the patient using crutches properly to achieve nonweight bearing).

*Epidemiology*

50 000 femoral neck fractures occur yearly in the UK; 20% of NHS orthopaedic beds are occupied by hip fracture patients alone as the length of stay is often protracted. Other lower limb fractures in the elderly are as common and as difficult as hip fractures (Fig. 133).

*Aetiology*

An ageing population, with falls and osteoporosis (which has an increasing incidence).

*Clinical features*

## Symptoms

Fracture symptoms of pain and loss of movement are present. It is sometimes difficult to obtain a clear history due to cognitive difficulties. It is essential to obtain details of previous medical and social history both to plan anaesthesia/surgery and also subsequent rehabilitation.

## Signs

Fracture signs (pain on movement, deformity, swelling) are present. It is essential to make careful assessment of cardiovascular and pulmonary systems to minimise anaesthetic risks (Fig. 134).

*Investigations*

For most patients undergoing operative treatment, FBC, U&Es, an ECG, group and save (or cross match) should be obtained. Consider obtaining a chest X-ray. Appropriate fracture X-rays are required for diagnosis and planning of treatment.

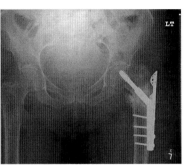 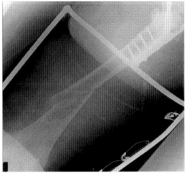

Fig. 133  This patient has a fracture below a previous implant (dynamic hip screw). This makes management more difficult as the choice of implants is limited by the other implant.

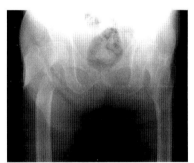 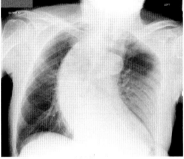

Fig. 134  This elderly patient has kyphoscoliosis and consequently reduced lung function and is at risk of perioperative problems.

*Management*

Management of these patients is multidisciplinary and demanding, because the physical (cardiovascular, pulmonary, renal) reserve of many patients is minimal. There are risks of:

- Cardiovascular problems: myocardial infarction, atrial fibrillation, fluid overload, or underperfusion
- Pulmonary problems: bronchopneumonia, pulmonary emboli (very common in older patients)
- Renal problems: renal failure, failure to excrete drugs such as morphine
- Cognitive problems: postoperative confusion (delirium, exacerbation of dementia)
- Metabolic problems: hyponatraemia (surgically induced inappropriate antidiuretic hormone)
- Pain problems: pain management is often difficult in these patients due to simultaneous fear of overdosage of opiates and the risks of NSAIDs in older patients; however, it is essential to control pain in order to reduce risks of postoperative immobility and also to reduce the risk of confusion

Management requires orthopaedic surgeons, specialists in elderly care, anaesthetists, physiotherapists, and skilled nursing and social workers all working together. Management of the above risks is important both in the acute perioperative phase and during rehabilitation. Rehabilitation requires mobilisation, psychological support (depression is common in elderly patients), and management of coincident medical conditions. Loss of previous mobility at this stage is common, which may mean that the patient cannot return to their original residence (where they may only just have been managing previously).

Decision making about fracture surgery is difficult in elderly patients—bone quality is poor, but most displaced lower limb fractures in elderly patients have operative treatment to permit early mobilisation and weight bearing (Fig. 135). Conversely, upper limb fractures may be more likely to be managed conservatively in the elderly, as functional demands are lower and risks of failure of fixation are higher than in younger patients (Fig. 136).

Finally, it is important to manage osteoporosis and address the causes of falls.

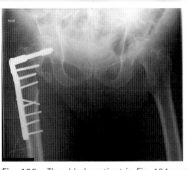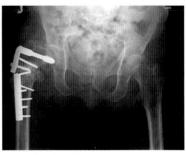

**Fig. 135** The elderly patient in Fig. 134 was operated on but the implant was insufficient to bear full weight as was required.

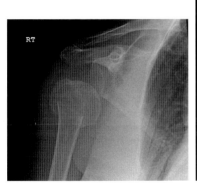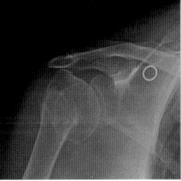

**Fig. 136** This fracture was treated nonoperatively—the relatively poor result was predicted but thought acceptable in view of the patient's age and other conditions.

# 38 Joint injuries

Joint injuries are common, but sometimes difficult to differentiate from fractures. They pose specific problems.

**Epidemiology**

Joint injuries are common in all age groups, but particularly frequent in young adults (where they may often be recurrent, such as shoulder or patellar dislocation or meniscal problems).

**Aetiology**

May occur due to injury (usually), predisposing anatomical abnormality, or joint laxity.

**Clinical features**

## Symptoms

These are typically pain and difficulty moving the joint. Neurovascular injuries are relatively common with joint injuries and require careful assessment. Later the patient may report recurrent mechanical symptoms such as locking or giving way.

## Signs

Joint injuries cause deformity, difficulty moving the joint, and distal neurovascular problems (paraesthesiae, loss of pulse). Swelling is often present, either within the joint (haemarthrosis or effusion) or surrounding oedema.

**Investigations**

X-rays in two planes are required. Occasionally diagnosis requires cross-sectional imaging (CT or MRI scan). It is important to ensure that you are dealing with a joint injury rather than a juxtarticular fracture before starting treatment such as manipulation. Injuries such as meniscal tears often require MRI scanning to define, as this is particularly useful for examining soft tissue injuries (Fig. 137)

**Management**

Dislocations require reduction of the dislocation (Fig. 138); recurrent dislocation may need reconstruction of the joint capsule. Injuries of intra-articular structures (for instance meniscal or cruciate ligament tears) may require surgery, which can often be done arthroscopically.

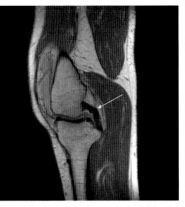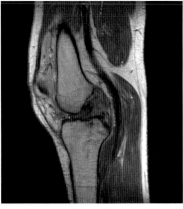

**Fig. 137** Patient with anterior cruciate ligament (ACL) injury after a ski accident. The posterior cruciate ligament (PCL) is clearly visible (arrow) but the ACL is not and has been injured.

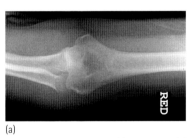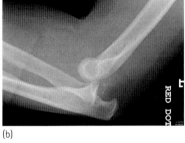

(a)                                              (b)

**Fig. 138** Anteroposterior (a) and lateral (b) view of an elbow dislocation.

## Shoulder dislocation

This the commonest joint dislocation and is particularly common in young adults, where it is frequently recurrent. The humeral head usually dislocates anteriorly and requires manipulation to reduce (Fig. 139). Shoulder dislocation is sometimes associated with axillary nerve palsy (which causes numbness in the 'regimental patch' area). This will usually recover spontaneously. Posterior dislocation also occurs (especially after electric shock or epileptic fit). This direction of dislocation may give anteroposterior X-rays that look almost normal. Both types of shoulder dislocation may require surgical stabilisation if recurrent.

## Elbow dislocation

This may be associated with brachial artery injury.

## Wrist sprain

Wrist sprains are very common; they usually resolve with no treatment but if severe pain and swelling are present consider damage to specific ligaments (most commonly the scapholunate ligament; damage to this causes a gap ('diastasis') to appear between scaphoid and lunate on X-ray) (Fig. 140).

## Hip dislocation

Hip dislocation is an uncommon injury, usually due to road traffic accidents (Fig. 141). Reduction of the joint is urgent due to the risk to the blood supply of the femoral head, and consequent avascular necrosis and hip arthritis.

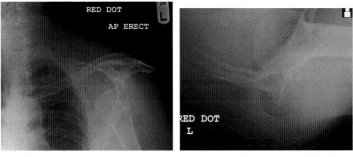

**Fig. 139** Patient with an anterior dislocation of the shoulder. Note the Hill Sach's deformity (fracture of the superior posterior aspect of the humeral head).

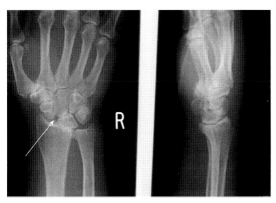

**Fig. 140** Patient with long-standing wrist problems—there is scapholunate diastasis (arrow) and she has developed osteoarthritis.

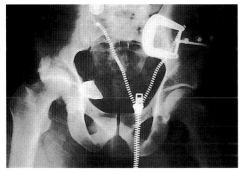

**Fig. 141** Patient with right hip dislocation. (Reproduced with permission from Andrew JG, Herrick AL, Marsh DR. Musculoskeletal Medicine and Surgery. Elsevier-Churchill Livingstone, Edinburgh, 2000.)

# Knee (tibiofemoral) dislocation

Knee dislocation is an uncommon injury; however, it must be treated urgently as there is a high risk of popliteal artery injury and disastrous ischaemia (Fig. 142 & 143). Management usually includes some form of arterial imaging.

# Patellar dislocation

Patellar dislocation is common in adolescents. It almost always involves the patella dislocating laterally. The problem may be recurrent and require surgery.

# Meniscal tear

Meniscal tears are a common problem, often due to injury (in younger patients) but may be due to degenerate meniscal changes (in older patients). They often cause locking of the knee (where the patient is unable to fully extend the knee), swelling (effusion), giving way, and joint line pain. The best signs are a block to full extension (compare the other side) and joint line tenderness. X-rays are usually normal, but an MRI scan may be helpful in diagnosis (Fig. 144). Treatment usually involves excision of the torn segment of meniscus or repair; both are usually achieved with use of an arthroscope (a telescope and associated fine instruments inserted into the joint via small incisions).

# Cruciate ligament injury

Anterior cruciate injury is the commonest. These are usually due to sporting injury—typically this causes immediate swelling in the joint due to haemarthrosis (unlike a meniscal tear where onset of swelling/effusion is over 24 hours as the meniscus does not have a blood supply). It is important to assess any damage to the collateral ligaments. Long-term problems may occur and patients often have recurrent giving way of the joint and sometimes a sensation of the joint 'coming out'. Treatment is by physiotherapy initially; surgical reconstruction of ligaments may prevent instability and giving way, and is often required to permit the patient to resume sports.

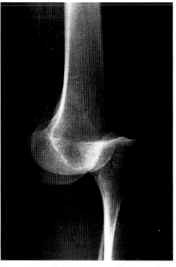
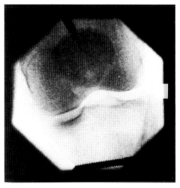

Figs. 142 and 143   X-ray of a knee dislocation. The second x-ray is of an angiogram after reduction which shows a complete block of the popliteal artery. (Reproduced with permission from Andrew JG, Herrick AL, Marsh DR. Musculoskeletal Medicine and Surgery. Elsevier-Churchill Livingstone, Edinburgh, 2000.)

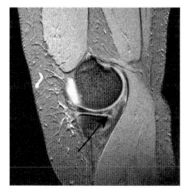

Fig. 144   MRI of a medial meniscal tear (arrow). (Reproduced with permission from Andrew JG, Herrick AL, Marsh DR. Musculoskeletal Medicine and Surgery. Elsevier-Churchill Livingstone, Edinburgh, 2000.)

## Ankle sprain

Ankle sprains are of variable severity. Most can be treated by elevation, pain relief, physiotherapy, and support by bandage or splint. A few patients have persistent symptoms of the joint giving way and require surgical reconstruction of the injured ligament. This is almost always the anterior talofibular ligament—patients have maximal pain and swelling just anterior to the lateral malleolus as opposed to over the bone (as would be the case in a lateral malleolus fracture).

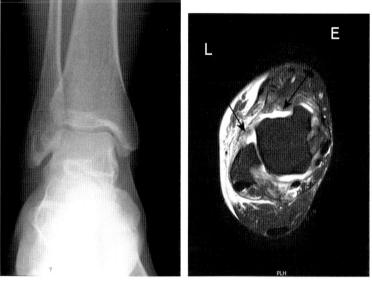

**Fig. 145** This patient has a sprained ankle. There is no abnormality seen on the x ray. However, on the MRI scan there is thinning of the anterior talo fibular ligament (L), and an effusion (E) in the ankle joint.

Soft tissue injuries may affect skin, nerve, vessels, tendon, or muscle. Management requires specific diagnosis and assessment; plastic surgeons are sometimes involved in the care of these patients, especially if microscope repair (of nerves or small blood vessels) is needed, or if there is extensive tissue loss.

*Aetiology*

Soft tissue injuries may arise due to injury (usually penetrating trauma—frequently lacerations with glass in the UK, gunshot wounds in the USA), but also almost spontaneously due to degenerative changes especially in tendons.

*Clinical features*

### Symptoms

These injuries may present with laceration and bleeding or loss of function (tendons, nerves). Closed soft tissue injury presents with sudden onset bruising and loss of power in the affected area of the limb.

### Signs

With lacerations assessment of distal neurovascular status is vital but difficult as patients may say sensation is still present even if the nerve is completely divided. It is best to compare sensation with that of the other side and ask if the sensation feels normal—if it does not the laceration should be explored. With a laceration a tendon injury is assessed as being present if there is limitation of movement of the joint served by the tendon. It is vital to assess for closed soft tissue injuries carefully. In particular, missed Achilles, quadriceps, and patellar tendon ruptures are common and these frequently result in litigation.

*Investigations*

X-rays should be taken if a laceration with glass has occurred, to ensure that no radiopaque glass is still in the wound (where it may cause further damage) (Fig. 146). The commonest way of further assessment of lacerations is surgical exploration under adequate anaesthetic (often using a tourniquet if the laceration is peripheral in the limb). Closed soft tissue injuries can often be assessed further by ultrasound examination; X-rays are not usually helpful. MRI scans may be useful.

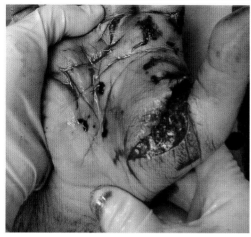

**Fig. 146** This patient has an unpleasant hand laceration sustained on glass.

*Management*   *Lacerations*   Explore to assess involvement of deep tissues; repair these and suture subcutaneous tissues and skin.

*Nerve injuries*   Penetrating injuries require detection (preoperative assessment and then surgical exploration). Nerves must be repaired accurately with fine sutures. Even then recovery is often very slow (axons regrow at 1mm per day) and function may be poor. Late results of these lesions (e.g. ulnar claw hand) are favourite cases in medical exams. Closed injuries may occur due to crush or stretching injury. Isolated closed injuries, such as radial nerve palsy due to leaving the arm hanging over a chair, should be treated expectantly (i.e. wait and see), but beware of vascular injuries at the same site. Multiple nerve injuries (e.g. brachial plexus injuries due to motorbike accidents) may be devastating and require surgery to obtain some improvement.

# Tendon lacerations

These are commonest at the hand and wrist, and are often due to cuts on glass (Fig. 147).

*Extensor tendons*   These require repair. Good results may be anticipated with lacerations over an area from the metacarpophalangeal joints proximally. Repair is more difficult over the finger due to the complex anatomy and the tendency for tendon to stick down to the underlying bone and limit movement.

*Flexor tendons*   These require repair. There is often coexistent nerve or vessel injury. Results are poor in the proximal part of the finger (two tendons in one flexor sheath).

# Tendon ruptures

*Biceps*   This usually occurs spontaneously in older patients, resulting in a 'Popeye' appearance of the biceps with a bulge due to rupture of the (proximal) long head attachment (Fig. 148). This is usually left untreated.

*Quadriceps/patella tendon ruptures*   These are usually spontaneous, sometimes occurring with athletic activity. A palpable gap in the tendon may be detected. It is essential to assess ability to straight leg raise in all knee injuries. If the patient is unable to do this, assess the continuity of the tendon with ultrasound; surgical repair should be undertaken if a rupture is present.

*Achilles tendon ruptures*   The tendo Achilles frequently ruptures in middle-aged and older patients who sometimes report a feeling of being hit on the back of the ankle during a game of squash or football. Examine for a gap in the tendon; surprisingly the patient is often still able to plantar flex the foot. It is essential to perform the Simmonds test (patient face down, feet extending beyond end of couch; squeeze both calves in turn—tendo Achilles injury results in the foot of the injured leg failing to plantar flex with this test). Management of tendo Achilles rupture is controversial—this may be by plaster in equinus (plantar flexion) or by surgical repair.

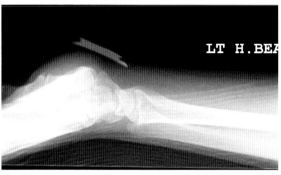

**Fig. 147** The large radio opaque foreign body (glass) was not immediately visible on clinical examination, but was obvious on x ray! It required removal at operation. A fragment of this size could easily cause further nerve or tendon damage if not detected and removed.

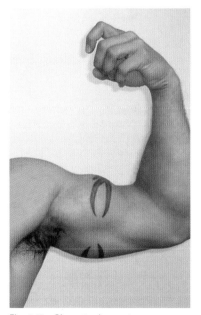

**Fig. 148** Biceps tendon rupture

**Benign hypermobility syndrome**

| | |
|---|---|
| *Definition* | The occurrence of musculoskeletal symptoms in hypermobile subjects in the absence of demonstrable systemic rheumatological disease. It is 'benign' in that life-threatening complications are not a feature. |
| *Epidemiology* | Generalised ligamentous laxity is common and is present in the order of 10% of healthy individuals, most of whom have no significant musculoskeletal symptoms. Hypermobility is especially common in children. |
| *Aetiology* | This is thought to be a genetically determined hereditable disorder of connective tissue. |
| *Clinical features* | Tests used to identify hypermobility are the ability to: |

* Appose the thumb to the flexor aspect of the forearm
* Passively dorsiflex the little finger (at the MCP joint) to 90° (Fig. 149c)
* Hyperextend the elbow beyond 10° (Fig. 149a)
* Hyperextend the knee beyond 10°
* Place the palms of the hand flat on the floor with the knees extended (Fig. 149b)

Joint hypermobility may be pauciarticular.

Common clinical features of hypermobility syndrome are arthralgia, myalgia, and back pain. There may be a low-grade synovitis. A number of extra-articular features may occur including hyperextensible skin.

| | |
|---|---|
| *Differential diagnosis* | Benign hypermobility syndrome must be distinguished from more severe hereditable disorders of connective tissue including: |

* Marfan's syndrome. Patients often have cardiac or ocular features, or a positive family history of Marfan's.
* Ehlers-Danlos syndrome type IV, in which associated vascular defects can lead to arterial rupture. There is a characteristic facies, marked bruising, and an 'aged' skin appearance.

| | |
|---|---|
| *Management* | The key points are patient education and physiotherapy (for muscle strengthening exercises and joint protection). |

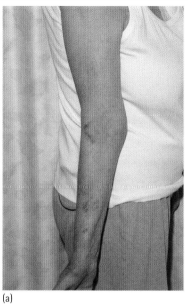

(a)

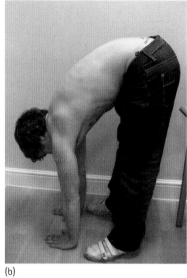

(b)

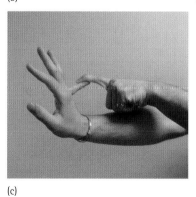

(c)

**Fig. 149** Hypermobile spine (a), hypermobile back (b), and hypermobility in little finger (c).

# ? Questions

**1.** This patient developed persistent, burning pain and swelling following a trivial injury.

a. What is the diagnosis?
b. What other symptoms is the patient likely to complain of?
c. What should you look for on examination?

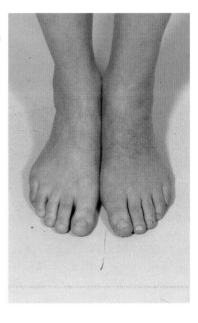

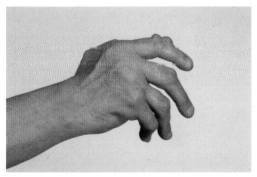

**2.** This patient has a chronic polyarthritis.

a. What is the diagnosis?
b. Describe the abnormalities?
c. What immunological test is likely to be positive?
d. What is the patient likely to complain of?

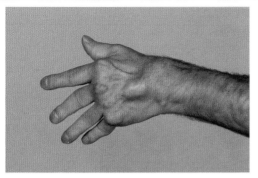

**3.** This patient has rheumatoid arthritis and complains of pain in her wrist. The key issue is whether there is active inflammation present.

*a.* What do you see on examination consistent with inflammation?
*b.* What might you feel consistent with inflammation?
*c.* If the joint is inflamed, how might movement be affected?

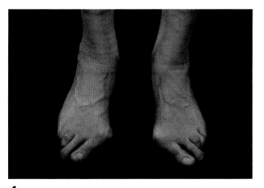

**4.** This patient has rheumatoid arthritis.

*a.* Describe the abnormalities.
*b.* What is the patient likely to complain of?
*c.* To whom should the patient be referred?

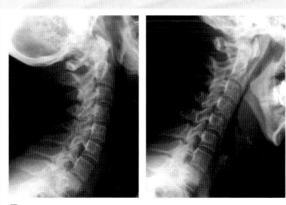

**5.** This patient with rheumatoid arthritis has a long history of neck pain and is about to have cardiac surgery. The anaesthetist has requested radiographs of the cervical spine (flexion and extension views).

*a.* Why have both flexion and extension views been requested?
*b.* What do the radiographs show?
*c.* What is the patient at risk of during intubation for general anaesthesia?

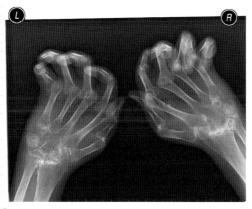

**6.** These radiographs are of a patient with polyarticular joint disease.

*a.* Describe the abnormalities.
*b.* What is the likely diagnosis?
*c.* Explain the basis of your diagnosis.

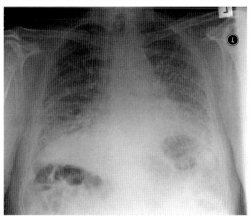

**7.** This is the chest X-ray of a patient who attends the rheumatology clinic. He/she is compaining of breathlessness.

*a.* Describe the abnormalities.
*b.* What is the main differential diagnosis?

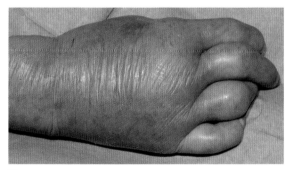

**8.** This patient with both osteoarthritis and gout has developed an extremely painful hand and wrist.

*a.* Describe the abnormalities.
*b.* What is the main clinical concern?
*c.* What is the single most important procedure/investigation?

**9.** This patient has rheumatoid arthritis and is having right ankle problems.

a. Describe the abnormalities.
b. What is a possible complication of rheumatoid nodules?
c. Which drug used in the treatment of rheumatoid arthritis can exacerbate the nodular component of the disease?

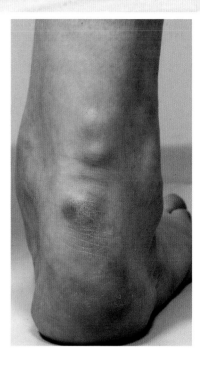

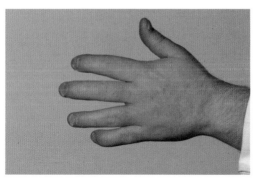

**10.** This patient complains of joint pain. The ESR and CRP are high, consistent with joint inflammation.

a. What is the diagnosis?
b. Describe the abnormalities.
c. Why is it important to examine his/her spine?
d. What might be an appropriate first choice of disease-modifying drug?

**11.** This patient complains of pain in the thumb.

a. What three abnormalities do you see?
b. What is the diagnosis?

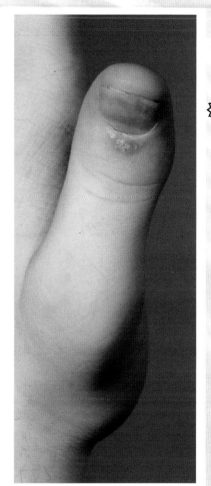

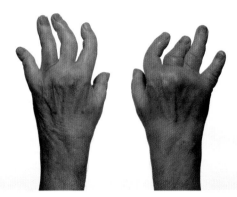

**12.** This patient has psoriatic arthritis and has developed 'arthritis mutilans', a form of destructive arthritis that can occur as part of the spectrum of psoriatic arthritis and also in patients with rheumatoid arthritis.

*a.* What do you see?
*b.* What would you expect to see on plain radiographs?

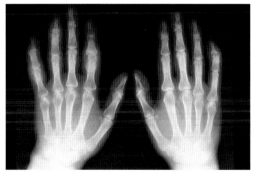

**13.** The complaint here was of painful, swollen fingers, troublesome for many years.

*a.* Describe the abnormalities.
*b.* What is the likely diagnosis?
*c.* Why are these *not* the hands of a patient with rheumatoid arthritis?

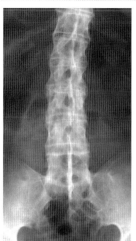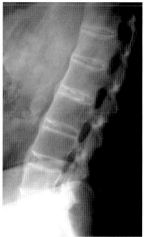

**14.** These radiographs are from a patient with back pain. On examination the spinal movements are reduced in all planes (flexion, extension, and lateral bending).

a. Describe the abnormalities.
b. What is the diagnosis?
c. At what time of day is his pain likely to be at its worst?

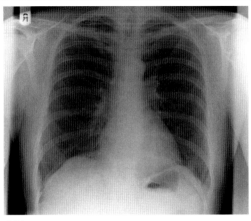

**15.** A young man with systemic lupus erythematosus (SLE) who is strongly antinuclear antibody positive attends the accident and emergency (A&E) department with a 12-hour history of left-sided pleuritic pain. He undergoes a detailed history and examination, and has blood tests and a chest X-ray, shown here.

*a.* What does the chest X-ray show?
*b.* What is the main differential diagnosis for the pleuritic pain?
*c.* Raised levels of which autoantibody are highly suggestive of active SLE?

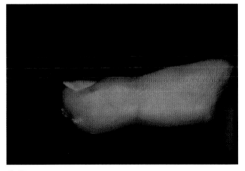

**16.** This patient complains of colour changes in her hands in the cold weather.

*a.* Describe the abnormalities that you see.
*b.* What is the diagnosis?
*c.* What other symptom is she very likely to have?

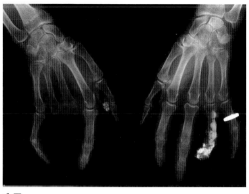

**17.** These are the hand radiographs of a patient with limited cutaneous systemic sclerosis.

*a.* What abnormalities do you see?
*b.* Why has she lost two fingers?
*c.* Which antibody is highly specific (but not sensitive) for limited cutaneous systemic sclerosis?

**18.** This patient with systemic sclerosis was admitted with vomiting and abdominal pain/distension.

*a.* What do you see?
*b.* Why has this developed?
*c.* What is a more common presentation of small bowel involvement in patients with systemic sclerosis?

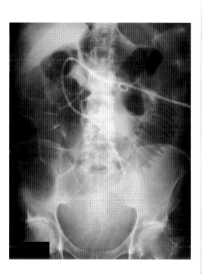

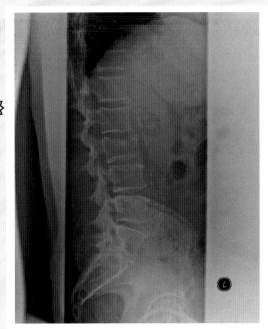

**19.** This female patient is complaining of low back pain.

*a.* What does the X-ray show?
*b.* What is the most likely cause?
*c.* What are the key aspects of management?

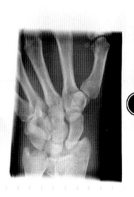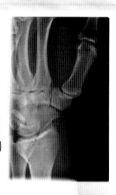

**20.** A 45-year-old female falls and sustains a radial fracture. She was surprised as she did not fall heavily. This is her first fracture.

*a.* What do you see on the X-ray?
*b.* What questions would you like to ask her to assess her osteoporosis risk?
*c.* Is there any further imaging you would like to arrange?

**21** This patient presented with acute knee pain and swelling. Polarising microscopy of the synovial fluid showed pyrophosphate crystals (weakly positively birefringent). The knee X-ray is shown.

a. What is the key abnormality?
b. What conditions could the chondrocalcinosis be secondary to and should be screened for?
c. What abnormalities in the biochemical profile would you be interested to look for in the search for an underlying cause of the pseudogout?

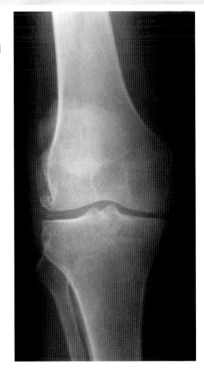

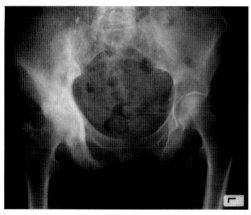

**22.** This patient complains of pain in the right hip/pelvis.

*a.* Describe the abnormality?
*b.* What is the likely diagnosis?
*c.* What abnormality would you expect to find on the biochemical profile?
*d.* What treatment would you recommend?

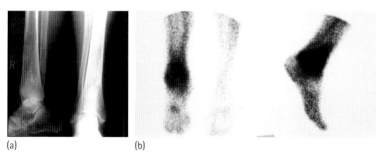

(a)                              (b)

**23.** This patient presented with a painful ankle and was feeling generally unwell with fever. Both the plain radiograph (a) and the isotope bone scan (b) are shown.

*a.* Describe the abnormalities on X-ray.
*b.* Describe the abnormalities on the isotope bone scan.
*c.* What is the likely diagnosis?
*d.* What treatment would you recommend?

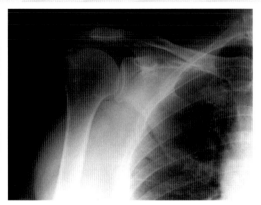

**24.** This is the radiograph of a patient complaining of a painful shoulder. She has a painful arc of abduction.

*a.* What do you see?
*b.* What is the most likely diagnosis?
*c.* What are the treatment options?

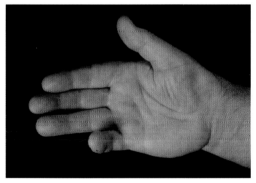

**25.** This patient complains of tingling in the fingers of the right hand. Thumb, index, and middle fingers are affected and the tingling tends to be worst in the early hours of the morning.

*a.* What is the most likely diagnosis?
*b.* What clinical signs (provocation tests) might be positive?
*c.* What investigation would help in confirming the diagnosis?
*d.* What possible underlying medical conditions should be considered?

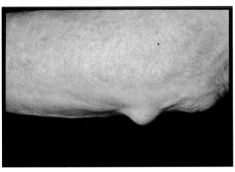

**26.** This patient complains of a lump at the elbow. On palpation, the lump is mobile and rubbery. There is a long history of joint complaints.

*a.* What is the lump?
*b.* What blood test is likely to be positive?
*c.* One year later, the patient has a chest X-ray and is noted to have a coin-shaped lesion. What is the differential diagnosis?

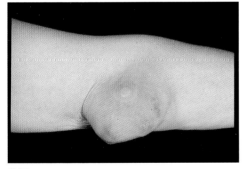

**27.** This patient with rheumatoid arthritis complains of elbow pain and a swelling 'behind' the elbow.

*a.* What do you see?
*b.* What is the diagnosis of the elbow lesion?
*c.* What treatment would you recommend?

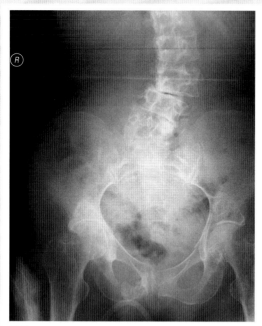

**28.** This is the X-ray of a patient who has back pain.

*a.* Describe the abnormalities.
*b.* Is the pain likely to be at its worst first thing in the morning or after activity?
*c.* In general terms, is there a relationship between these types of abnormality and the severity of back pain?

**29.** This is an X-ray of the lumbosacral spine

a. What is the abnormality?
b. What might the patient complain of?
c. What are the possible causes of this abnormality.

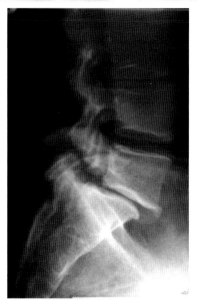

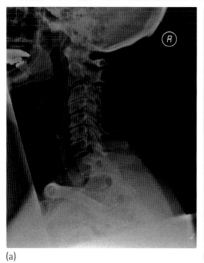
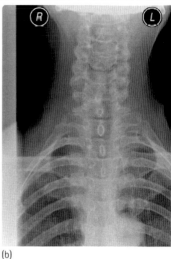

(a)                                      (b)

**30.** This elderly patient complains of neck pain. She has (a) lateral and (b) anteroposterior X-rays taken.

a. Describe the abnormalities.
b. What is the diagnosis?
c. If she develops pain and/or paraesthesia down either left or right upper limb, and after careful assessment these symptoms are thought to be radicular, what further imaging might you request?

**31.** This patient has a very stiff neck. He also has low back pain.

a. Describe the abnormalities.
b. What is the diagnosis?
c. At what time of day are his symptoms likely to be worst?

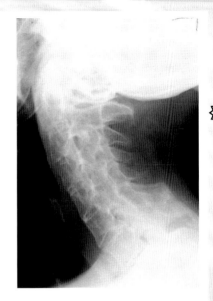

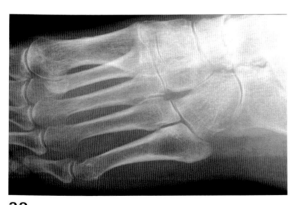

**32.** This patient complains of pain in the mid-foot.

a. Describe the abnormalities.
b. What is the diagnosis?
c. What is the first-line management?

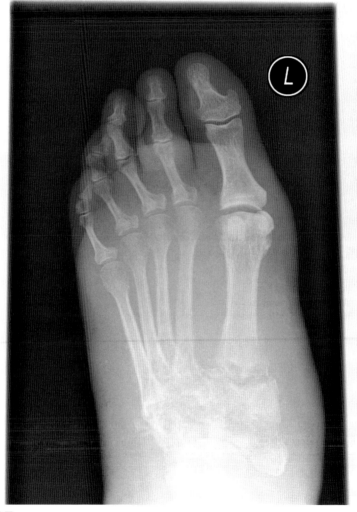

**37.** This is the X-ray of a patient complaining of a swollen foot and ankle, which were not particularly painful.

a. Describe the abnormalities.
b. What is the most likely diagnosis?
c. What is the most likely underlying general medical condition?

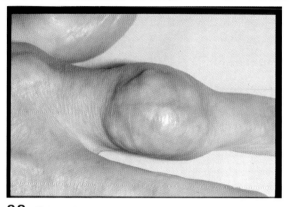

**38.** This patient presents with a firm lump at the index PIP joint.

*a.* Describe the abnormality.
*b.* What is the likely diagnosis?
*c.* What blood test is likely to be abnormal?

**39.** This patient has a spinal deformity.

*a.* Describe the deformity.
*b.* When leg length discrepancy occurs secondary to a fixed scoliosis, Is this a true or apparent leg length discrepancy?

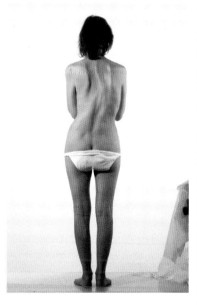

**40.** This patient has long-standing knee pain, especially on the left. His walking is severely limited.

a. Describe the deformity of the left knee.
b. What is the likely underlying disease process?
c. What are the likely findings on X-ray of the left knee?

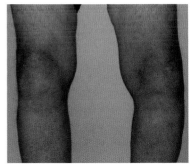

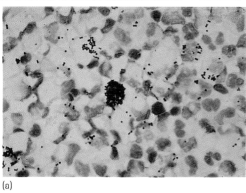

(a)

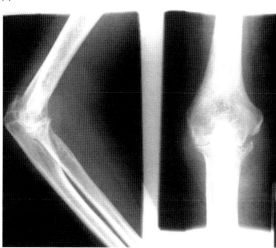

(b)

**41.** This patient has long-standing arthritis of the elbow. There has been a sudden exacerbation of her symptoms and she has become systemically unwell. The illustration shows a microscope picture of a joint aspirate (a) and X-rays of her elbow (b). (Part a reproduced with permission from Andrew JG, Herrick AL, Marsh DR. Musculoskeletal Medicine and Surgery. Elsevier–Churchill Livingstone, Edinburgh, 2000.)

*a.* What does the joint aspirate show?
*b.* What type of arthritis do you think she has?
*c.* What do you think caused this patient's septic arthritis?

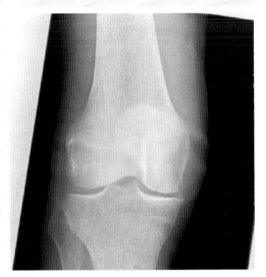

**42.** This 67-year-old patient has developed recurrent pain in the knee. It is principally at the lateral side. Serum urate is normal.

a. What is the likely cause of this joint disease?
b. What would you expect to find on polarized light microscopy of a joint aspirate?
c. The patient has severe pain and inflammation in the knee. How can you treat this?

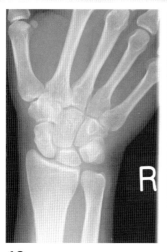 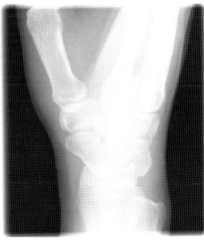

**43.** This patient has had a fall and complains of pain in the wrist. She is tender over the dorsum of the wrist and in the anatomical snuff box.

a. What diagnoses would you consider?
b. How would you treat her and why?
c. After 2 weeks she is still very tender in the anatomical snuff box and wrist movement is painful. X-rays are unchanged. What would you do now?

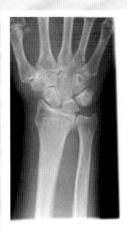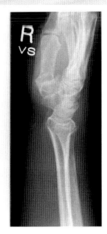

**44.** This 45-year-old patient has a fall and complains of severe pain in the wrist and paraesthesia in the radial side of the hand.

a. What is the diagnosis?
b. How would you treat this?
c. The paraesthesiae persist after the fracture has been treated. What treatment should be considered?

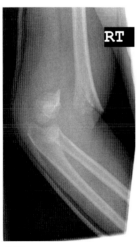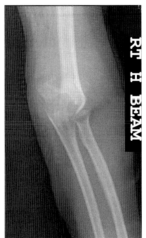

**45.** This patient aged 6 years has fallen on his outstretched arm.

a. What injury can you see?
b. What treatment would you recommend and why?
c. What other problems are common after this injury?

**46.** This patient has sustained an injury of the finger and presents to A&E.

a. What will you find on examination of this patient's finger?
b. How would you describe the X-ray on the phone to your supervising consultant?
c. What treatment would you recommend?

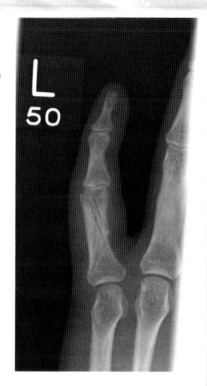

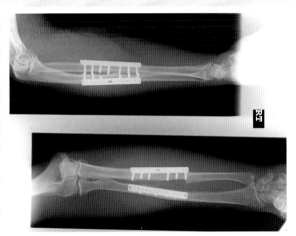

**47.** This patient had a fall and now complains of pain in his forearm. He had previously sustained a radius and ulna fracture some 15 years previously.

a. What treatment had been provided previously for the initial forearm fracture?
b. What is the current diagnosis?
c. Why has this occurred?

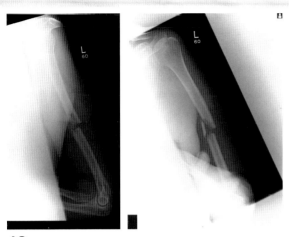

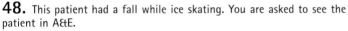

**48.** This patient had a fall while ice skating. You are asked to see the patient in A&E.

a. In which area would you test sensation to see if nerve injury had occurred?
b. The patient is treated with a 'U slab' cast which uses the weight of the cast to act as traction, and a sling. What are the pros and cons of plaster treatment of fractures?
c. The fracture fails to heal after 4 months treatment and is still very mobile. What would you recommend now?

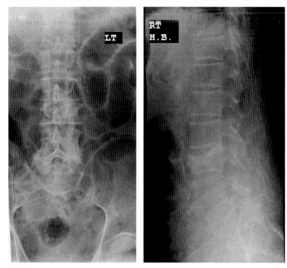

**49.** This 84-year-old patient presents with upper lumbar back pain for the last week. The X-rays are as shown. She is otherwise well with no significant medical history.

a. What is the likely diagnosis?
b. She has been in bed for a week. Should you advise mobilisation or further rest due to the risk of nerve injury?
c. What other investigations should be considered?

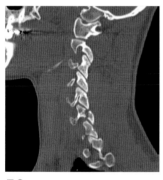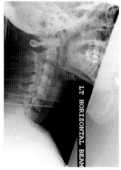

**50.** This patient has been injured in a road traffic accident and complains of neck pain. He cannot recall the exact mechanism of injury. There is no abnormal neurology. X-rays and CT scans of the cervical spine are shown.

a. What injury can you see on these X-rays?
b. How would you manage this?
c. What would you expect if there was a neurological injury at this level?

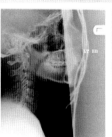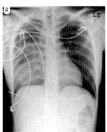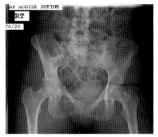

**51.** This patient is brought to A&E after a road traffic accident. As part of the standard work up of potentially multiply injured patients, X-rays of chest, cervical spine, and pelvis are obtained.

*a.* What comment would you make about the cervical spine X-ray?
*b.* What abnormality can you see on the pelvic X-ray?
*c.* Name three nonbony structures that may have been injured.

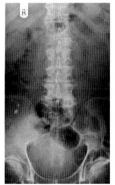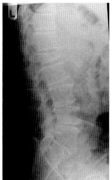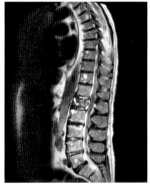

**52.** This 75-year-old patient presents with weakness in both lower limbs and incontinence. He also has had back pain for some months. He has no known other diseases. The X-rays and MRI of his lumbar spine are shown.

*a.* What is your provisional diagnosis?
*b.* How would you investigate this?
*c.* What treatment is possible?

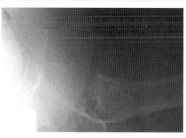 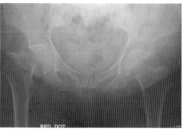

**53.** An 84-year-old lady presents following a fall at home. An anteroposterior (AP) X-ray of her hips and a lateral X-ray of the right hip are shown. She is otherwise well.

a. What sort of hip fracture has occurred? What are the major risks to the hip with this fracture?
b. How would you treat this?
c. How would you treat this in a 40-year-old patient?

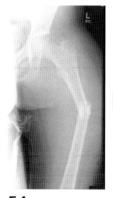 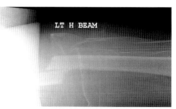

**54.** This 14-year-old patient has sustained the injury shown.

a. Why do you think this fracture has occurred?
b. How would you treat this fracture?
c. How would you treat this fracture in a 2-year-old child?

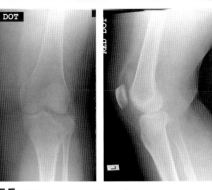
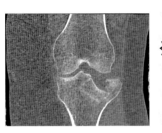

**55.** This 22-year-old patient has sustained the closed knee injury shown on the X-rays and CT scans. It is her only injury.

*a.* How would you treat the patient in A&E?
*b.* What are the long-term risks of this fracture and how can the risks be minimised?

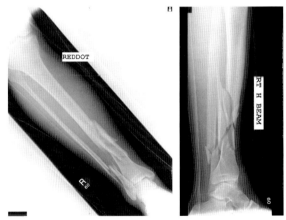

**56.** Your patient has sustained the closed tibial fracture shown.

*a.* What is the most likely method of treatment of this fracture?
*b.* What would the risks be if this was an open (compound) tibial fracture?
*c.* The patient had his fracture treated 1 day ago. You are asked to see him due to severe pain in the leg, which has deteriorated over the last 12 hours. The leg is rather swollen. What would you do?

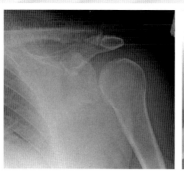 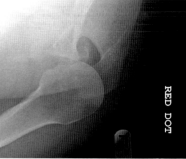

RED DOT

**57.** This epileptic patient complains of shoulder pain after a fit. He tells you that this has happened several times before.

a. What is the diagnosis?
b. What is the commonest complication of this injury?
c. How should this be treated?

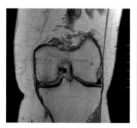 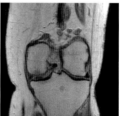 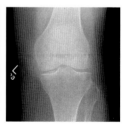

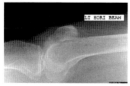

**58.** This patient has sustained a knee injury that resulted in severe swelling of the knee after about 12 hours.

a. What is the most likely cause of the swelling?
b. What does the MRI scan show?
c. What are the problems that follow this type of injury?

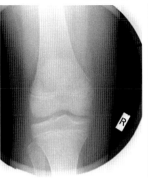
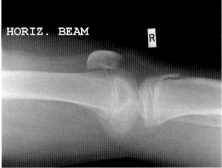
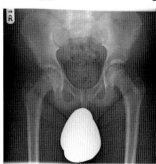
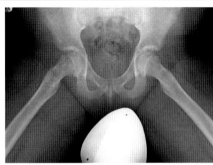

**59.** This 12-year-old child complains of right knee pain for 3 weeks. In the last week he has also had right hip pain and started to limp.

a. What is the likely diagnosis?
b. What are the risks if this is not detected?
c. What else should you enquire after and seek on examination and X-rays?

**60.** This 30-year-old alcoholic patient who takes oral steroids for asthma complains of severe hip pain on the right. The X-ray is as shown.

a. What is the most likely diagnosis?
b. How should this be investigated?

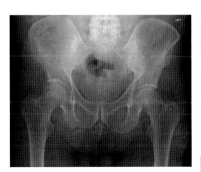

(Figure reproduced with permission from Andrew JG, Herrick AL, Marsh DR. Musculoskeletal Medicine and Surgery. Elsevier–Churchill Livingstone, Edinburgh, 2000.)

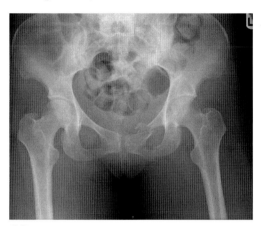

**62.** This 70-year-old patient has fallen and cannot walk.

*a.* What injury has the patient sustained?
*b.* Other than the initial treatment what action should be taken?

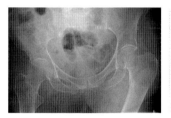 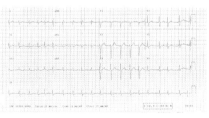

**63.** This patient has sustained the injury shown. The patient's electrocardiogram (ECG) obtained in A&E is also shown.

*a.* What injury has the patient sustained?
*b.* What does the ECG show? How does this and the associated treatment affect your treatment plans?
*c.* Two days after surgery her urea and electrolytes (U&Es) are: Na 122 mmol/L; K 3.3 mmol/L; Urea 3.6 mmol/L; Creatinine 77 μmol/L. Preoperatively her U&Es were normal, although she was on bendroflumethiazide. Her urine looks concentrated. What is the cause of this problem and how should you treat it?

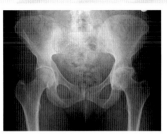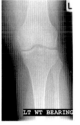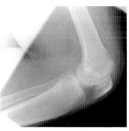

**64.** This 55-year-old patient has left knee pain and a limp.

*a.* What is the likely cause of the pain?

*b.* What conservative treatments would you recommend?

*c.* What surgical treatments are possible? What are the risks and benefits?

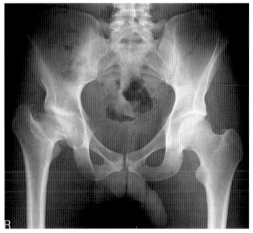

**65.** This 25-year-old patient had problems with the right hip as a child (aged 6 to 10) and now presents with pain and shortening of the leg.

*a.* What is the most likely diagnosis of the condition as a child?

*b.* What would the differential diagnosis include?

*c.* What treatment would you recommend now?

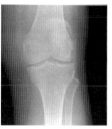
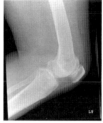
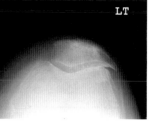

**66.** This patient has knee pain on stairs and kneeling.

*a.* Which part of the knee do you think is the problem?
*b.* What abnormalities can you see on the X-rays?
*c.* What treatment would you recommend?

**67.** This patient complains of a deformed foot and difficulty with footwear.

*a.* What do you think is the likely diagnosis?
*b.* What treatment would you recommend?
*c.* If surgery was considered, what risks would you warn the patient about?

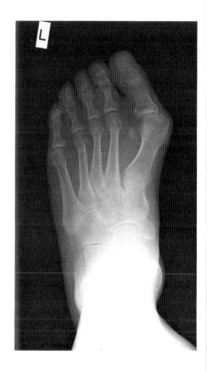

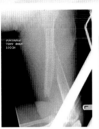 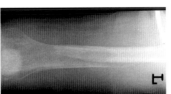 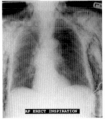

**68.** This 70-year-old patient has the injuries shown after a road traffic accident. You see the patient in the A&E department.

a. What initial steps would you take in managing this patient?
b. What abnormality can you see on the chest X-ray? What should be done?
c. How would you manage the open femoral fracture?

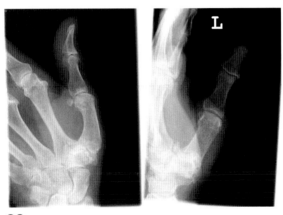

**69.** This patient has pain at the base of the left thumb.

a. What do you think is the responsible pathology?
b. What treatment would you recommend?

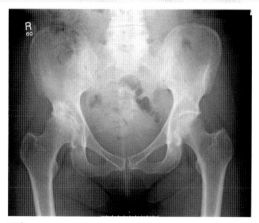

**70.** This patient has right hip pain.

*a.* What radiological signs can you see at the right hip? What is the likely diagnosis?

# Answers

**1.**
a. Complex regional pain syndrome type I (also commonly called reflex sympathetic dystrophy). Several other terms have been used to describe this condition including 'algodystrophy' and 'Sudeck's atrophy'.
b. The patient may complain of changes in colour (the affected extremity may be red, blue, or mottled at variable times), in temperature, and in sweating.
c. The limb is usually extremely tender with allodynia (a stimulus such as light touch which would normally be painless is painful). Swelling (as shown here) is common. Colour, temperature, and/or sweating changes may be present. There may be increased hair growth (as shown here). Rarely a patient will progress to dystrophic change, contractures, and/or tremor.

**2.**
a. Rheumatoid arthritis.
b. Ulnar deviation and flexion at the MCP joints. Rheumatoid nodules overlying the index finger PIP joint. Wasting of the small muscles of the hand. The flexed position at the ring and little MCP joints (and absence of visible extensor tendons to these fingers) suggest extensor tendon rupture.
c. Rheumatoid factor, especially because the patient has rheumatoid nodules. Rheumatoid factor can be measured in a number of different ways, for example, by the sheep cell agglutination test (SCAT).
d. Pain, stiffness (especially in the morning), swelling, and symptoms of loss of function, e.g. difficulty with fine finger movements.

**3.**
a. Swelling, affecting the wrist and the extensor tendon compartment. There is also muscle wasting.
b. Tenderness and 'boggy' synovial swelling.
c. Movement will probably be painful and restricted.

**4.**
a. Hallux valgus, with flexion at the PIP joints (especially the 3rd left). The flexion at the PIP joints typically occurs in association with subluxation at the MTP joints.
b. Forefoot pain on walking. The patient may describe as if 'walking on pebbles'.
c. A podiatrist (chiropodist). If the patient continues to have severe pain despite appropriate orthotic/footwear provision then surgical referral may be indicated.

**5.**
a. To look for instability. Atlantoaxial subluxation will be more evident on the flexion view, because the normal close apposition of the odontoid peg to the anterior arch of the atlas is lost.

b. Atlantoaxial subluxation.

c. Damage to the spinal cord.

**6.**
a. There is advanced bilateral symmetrical erosive arthropathy of the carpus with joint space loss and fusion of the midcarpal joints. There is marked subluxation at the MCP joints with ulnar deviation.

b. Rheumatoid arthritis.

c. The diagnosis is made on the basis of: (1) the distribution of the joint disease (wrists, MCPs, and PIPs); and (2) the typical radiographic changes with periarticular bone loss and erosion and (in this case of advanced disease) fusion.

**7.**
a. Bilateral interstitial shadowing, most pronounced at the lung bases.

b. Pulmonary fibrosis related to rheumatoid arthritis (rheumatoid lung disease), methotrexate (or other drug-induced) pneumonitis, infection (including opportunistic, because many patients with inflammatory arthritis or connective tissue disease are on immunosuppressant treatment), cardiac failure.

**8.**
a. The hand and wrist are swollen and erythematous. The likelihood (although not possible to state from the photograph) is that they will be very tender and painful to move.

b. That the joint is septic. The other possibility is that this is a severe exacerbation of gout.

c. To aspirate the joint and send the fluid for an urgent gram stain and also (less urgent) for crystal examination using a polarising microscope. Blood cultures should also be sent (sometimes the organism is isolated from the blood but not from the synovial fluid).

**9.**
a. The ankle is swollen and there are nodules in the area of the Achilles tendon. Rheumatoid nodules are found more commonly at the elbow but may occur elsewhere, for example, over pressure points including the Achilles tendon and sacrum.

b. The nodules can ulcerate and can be difficult to heal.

c. Methotrexate.

**10.**
a. Psoriatic arthritis.

b. Nail changes and swelling of the DIP joints (especially index and little fingers). These DIP joints will probably be tender, in contrast to the situation in osteoarthritis, when DIP swelling is usually nontender (and hard).

c. There may be involvement of the axial skeleton.

d. Methotrexate or ciclosporin are likely to have beneficial effects on both the skin and joint disease.

**11.**
a. (i) Swelling of the thumb MCP (and probably also of the IP) joint
   (ii) A small plaque of psoriasis
   (iii) Nail changes of psoriasis

b. Psoriatic arthritis.

**12.** *a.* Deformity with shortening ('telescoping') of several of the fingers, especially the right middle finger. Nail changes of psoriasis can be seen in the left middle and ring fingers.

*b.* A severe, erosive, destructive arthritis with 'pencil and cup' deformities.

**13.** *a.* (i) Soft tissue swelling of the left index and little PIP joints
(ii) Erosive change of several of the DIP joints and of the left index PIP
(iii) Acro-osteolysis (resorption of the terminal phalanges) of several fingers
(iv) New bone formation best seen in the proximal phalanges of the left index and little fingers, suggestive of an enthesopathy
The changes are asymmetrical.

*b.* These appearances suggest a seronegative arthritis, most likely psoriatic arthritis.

*c.* In rheumatoid arthritis, symmetrical changes are usually seen at the MCP, PIP joints, and wrists. The DIP joints are spared.

**14.** *a.* The anteroposterior view shows a 'dagger' spine and fused sacroiliac joints. The lateral view shows a 'bamboo' spine.

*b.* Ankylosing spondylitis (long-standing disease with sacroiliac and spinal fusion).

*c.* First thing in the morning. Ankylosing spondylitis is an inflammatory joint disease and so (unlike 'mechanical' back pain) is worst after inactivity, and is eased by movement.

**15.** *a.* The chest X-ray is normal.

*b.* (i) Serositis as part of the SLE disease process
(ii) Infection, including opportunistic (patients with SLE are prone to infection as they are often immunosuppressed as a result of their disease and/or their treatment)
(iii) Pulmonary embolism (especially likely if the patient has an antiphospholipid syndrome)

*c.* Antibodies to double-stranded DNA. High titres suggest active disease.

**16.** *a.* Calcinosis and a telangiectasis.

*b.* Limited cutaneous systemic sclerosis (previously often termed CREST—calcinosis, Raynaud's, oesophageal dysmotility, sclerodactyly, telangiectases).

*c.* Difficulty swallowing and/or heartburn, due to oesophageal dysmotility/reflux.

**17.** *a.* (i) Subcutaneous calcinosis of the left ring finger (very extensive) and of the right thumb.
(ii) Loss of the right middle and ring fingers (amputated at the level of the MCP joint).
(iii) Flexion contractures of the fingers (commonly seen in patients with systemic sclerosis).

b. Raynaud's phenomenon in patients with systemic sclerosis can be very severe, and most probably she developed critical ischaemia, in association with digital ulceration (possibly overlying an area of calcinosis). Gangrene and osteomyelitis can occur and can be very difficult to treat. A minority of patients require amputation.

c. Anticentromere antibody. In the order of 50% of patients with limited cutaneous systemic sclerosis are anticentromere antibody positive.

**18.** a. Distended bowel loops. The valvulae conniventes of the small bowel go all the way across the bowel whereas in the large bowel the haustra do not go completely across. There is a feeding line in situ. This bowel distension will have resulted in an intestinal pseudo-obstruction.

b. Dysmotility of the small bowel. In systemic sclerosis the whole of the bowel can become involved, and a minority of patients develop intestinal failure.

c. Weight loss and steattorhoea, usually a result of small bowel bacterial overgrowth (which in turn results from stasis in the small intestine).

**19.** a. Wedge compression fracture of L2. The vertebral body of L2 shows anterior compression which is greater than 20% loss in height compared to posterior body.

b. Osteoporosis.

c. (i) Establish the underlying cause of the osteoporosis. While is may be postmenopausal there could be other causes, e.g. myeloma and osteomalacia. Therefore, check a full blood count, ESR, biochemistry screen, and protein electrophoresis.

(ii) Lifestyle measures, e.g. stop smoking, exercise, adequate calcium intake.

(iii) Drug treatment, for example, calcium and vitamin D, bisphosphonates, selective oestrogen receptor modulators.

**20.** a. A comminuted fracture of distal radius with extension of the fracture line across the articular surface.

b. (i) Has she reached the menopause? If so, when, and did she have a hysterectomy? Has she had any ovarian surgery?

(ii) Does she have an adequate calcium intake?

(iii) Does she smoke?

(iv) Is there a family history of osteoporosis?

(v) Does she have any medical conditions (e.g. thyroid disease) or is she on any drug treatment (e.g. prednisolone) that could reduce bone density.

c. Measurement of bone density, probably by dual X-ray absorptiometry (DEXA).

**21.** a. Chondrocalcinosis. There is a line of calcification across both the lateral and medial menisci.

b. These include hyperparathyroidism and haemochromatosis.

c. The plasma calcium and phosphate. In hyperparathyroidism the calcium will be high and the phosphate low.

**22.** *a.* There is expansion of most of the right hemipelvis and of the femoral head with sclerosis.

    *b.* Paget's disease.

    *c.* The alkaline phosphatase will be high.

    *d.* Bisphosphonates are most commonly used in the treatment of symptomatic Paget's disease. Calcitonin is also used, but less frequently.

**23.** *a.* The plain film shows a lucent lesion of the distal tibia (just above the line of the physis) with well-defined sclerotic margins, typical of a Brodie's abscess (chronic bone infection).

    *b.* The isotope bone scan shows generalised increased uptake in the region of the distal tibia.

    *c.* Osteomyelitis.

    *d.* Six weeks' antibiotics (preferably guided by the organism isolated from pus or bone biopsy). Usually the first 2 weeks' antibiotic treatment is given intravenously. Surgery may also be indicated.

**24.** *a.* Calcification in the supraspinatus tendon.

    *b.* Calcific tendonitis

    *c.* Physiotherapy, NSAIDs and injection of the subacromial bursa with local anaesthetic and long-acting steroid are all possible options singly or in combination. If things do not settle then surgery may be indicated.

**25.** *a.* Carpal tunnel syndrome. There is wasting of the thenar eminence.

    *b.* Tinel's test and Phalen's test.

    *c.* Nerve conduction studies.

    *d.* Carpal tunnel syndrome commonly occurs in patients with inflammatory arthritis, due to compression of the median nerve by synovial hypertrophy at the wrist. However, here there is no obvious joint swelling to suggest inflammatory arthritis. Other conditions in which carpal tunnel syndrome occurs include pregnancy, hypothyroidism, and diabetes.

**26.** *a.* A rheumatoid nodule.

    *b.* Testing for rheumatoid factor. Patients with nodular rheumatoid arthritis are usually strongly rheumatoid factor positive.

    *c.* The main concern regarding a coin-shaped lesion on X-ray is a bronchial carcinoma. However, in a patient with nodular rheumatoid this could be a rheumatoid nodule.

**27.** *a.* Swelling of the olecranon bursa, with lesions within the bursa, and some erythema.

    *b.* Olecranon bursitis, with rheumatoid nodules within the bursa (although it is difficult to be sure about the nodules without being able to palpate these). The erythema is of concern, suggesting that there might be infection of the bursa.

c. Because of the size of the bursa (and the concern that this might be infected) the bursa should be aspirated and the fluid sent to microbiology. The plaster suggests that aspiration has already been performed. An NSAID will provide some symptomatic relief. Infection should be treated with antibiotics. In some cases of refractory bursitis, surgical excison may be indicated.

**28.** *a.* There is a scoliosis concave to the right. This is secondary to 'degenerative' spinal disease. There is marked mid-lumbar scoliosis with lateral subluxation of L3 on L4.

*b.* After activity. The pain felt is likely to be 'mechanical' and exacerbated by activities such as walking and bending.

*c.* There is no good relationship between the severity of 'degenerative' radiographic changes and the severity of pain—patients with severe changes on X-ray may have no symptoms and, conversely, patients with severe symptoms may have very little in the way of radiographic change.

**29.** *a.* Spondylolisthesis (forward displacement of one vertebra on another) of L5 on S1, associated with a defect in the pars interarticularis of L5).

*b.* Low back pain. Because of the slip, there is a possibility that there may be neurological compromise of the cauda equina.

*c.* Possible causes are 'degenerative', congenital, and traumatic.

**30.** *a.* The changes are those of cervical spondylosis, with loss of disc space and anterior osteophytes especially at the C3/4, C5/6, and C6/7 levels.

*b.* Cervical spondylosis.

*c.* An MR scan, looking for any compromise of the exiting nerve roots.

**31.** *a.* This cervical spine X-ray shows fusion of the anterior and posterior elements.

*b.* The appearances are very suggestive of ankylosing spondylitis, or one of the other spondyloarthropathies.

*c.* Most patients with ankylosing spondylitis feel most stiff first thing in the morning.

**32.** *a.* Loss of joint space, juxta-articular sclerosis, and osteophytes of the talonavicular joint.

*b.* Osteoarthritis of the talonavicular joint.

*c.* Analgesia and referral to podiatry for advice regarding footwear/orthotics.

**33.** *a.* The knees are diffusely swollen (especially the left).

*b.* The knee is likely to be warm and the swelling is likely to be tender and boggy (suggestive of synovitis). Also, there is likely to be a large joint effusion and so there will be a positive patellar tap.

*c.* Knee movement is likely to be painful and restricted.

**31.** *a.* There is swelling of the DIP joints and of the index and ring PIP joints (Heberden's and Bouchard's nodes). There is deformity at the index and little DIP joints.

*b.* The swellings are likely to be hard (bony) and nontender.

*c.* Osteoarthritis.

**35.** *a.* There is swelling of the prepatellar bursa, seen on both the frontal and lateral views.

*b.* Prepatellar bursitis. There is no obvious erythema and so this is unlikely to be infected.

*c.* In monoarthritis (or if the knee is swollen in an inflammatory polyarthritis such as rheumatoid), the knee is diffusely swollen and tender. If there is fluid in the knee there will probably be a positive patellar tap. In contrast, in prepatellar bursitis shown here, the swelling is confined to the prepatellar bursa, which will probably be fluctuant.

**36.** *a.* Typically the fingers go white (ischaemic phase), then blue (deoxygenation phase), then red (reperfusion phase).

*b.* It is important to determine whether the Raynaud's phenomenon is primary (idiopathic) or secondary to an underlying cause (e.g. a connective tissue disease). Therefore, a full history and examination are essential. The usual screening investigations include a full blood count, ESR, antinuclear antibody, and (if available) nailfold capillaroscopy (looking for capillary enlargement and areas of avascularity).

*c.* Management depends on severity. Many patients will respond to conservative measures alone (including keeping warm and stopping smoking). If these are not sufficient then vasodilatory therapy, for example with a calcium channel blocker, may be indicated.

**37.** *a.* There is gross destructive change with dislocation of the 2nd, 3rd and 4th tarsometatarsal joints.

*b.* A Charcot joint (characterised by gross destructive change).

*c.* Diabetes.

**38.** *a.* There is a periarticular swelling overlying the index PIP joint (dorsal aspect). The overlying skin is shiny and there is a yellowish discolouration beneath.

*b.* Tophaceous gout. This is a large tophus. There may well be tophi elsewhere, and on radiographs there may be erosive change at the PIP joint as the joint is likely to be involved.

*c.* The urate level will almost certainly be high.

**39.** *a.* There is a thoracic scoliosis, concave to the left.

*b.* Apparent—fixed scoliosis can result in an apparent leg length discrepancy, i.e. one leg appears shorter than the other, because of the resulting pelvic tilt. However, there is no real discrepancy—when each leg is measured from the anterior superior iliac spine to the medial malleolus they are of equal length. Conversely, a true leg length discrepancy can give rise to a compensatory scoliosis. In the example shown here, there is no apparent leg length discrepancy, because there is no pelvic tilt.

**40.** *a.* There is a varus deformity
   *b.* Osteoarthritis. Severe osteoarthritis of the knee can typically result in a varus deformity, due to loss of the medial joint space.
   *c.* Plain radiographs are likely to show loss of joint space (especially medially), subchondral sclerosis, osteophytes, and subchondral cysts.

**41.** *a.* This shows gram positive organisms; this is septic arthritis.
   *b.* She has rheumatoid arthritis. There is juxta-articular osteopenia, an obvious severe deformity of the elbow, minimal osteophytes, and fairly uniform loss of joint space. Soft tissue swelling due to synovitis is also sometimes present.
   *c.* Rheumatoid arthritis patients have damaged joints and are often on drugs that cause immune dysfunction, both of which predispose to septic arthritis. Septic arthritis is consequently common.

**42.** *a.* The presence of chondrocalcinosis (calcification of the articular cartilage and meniscus) strongly suggests that this is pseudogout (pyrophosphate crystal arthropathy).
   *b.* The aspirate of a joint with pseudogout would be expected to show pyrophosphate crystals, which are weakly positively birefringent on polarized light microscopy.
   *c.* Initial treatment is with NSAIDs. If severe pain persists the pain and inflammation can usually be controlled by injection of local anaesthetic and long-acting corticosteroid.

**43.** *a.* There is no sign of a distal radial fracture. Given the location of tenderness, the possibility of a scaphoid fracture should be considered; however, the most likely diagnosis remains a wrist sprain (soft tissue injury)
   *b.* Because of the possibility of a scaphoid fracture she should have a scaphoid cast for an initial period of 2 weeks and then be reassessed. It is unwise to leave someone with a suspected scaphoid

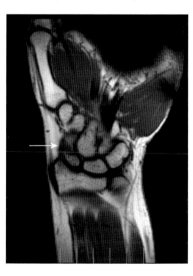

fracture without immobilisation because of the risk of patients developing a nonunion if a fracture is not immobilised.

c. There is still a possibility of a scaphoid fracture despite the second normal X-ray. The best investigation is an MRI scan. The scan showed the presence of a fracture across the waist of the scaphoid and a further period of immobilisation was required.

**44.** a. The patient has a displaced intra-articular distal radial fracture. The likely cause of the paraesthesia is acute carpal tunnel syndrome (median nerve compression) due to displacement and bleeding and swelling into the carpal tunnel.

b. The initial treatment is to reduce the fracture under anaesthetic. Most surgeons would now fix the fracture with plate or wire fixation, as it is important for wrist function for the anatomy of the distal radius to be accurately restored both to ensure adequate grip and prevent arthritis.

c. Early surgical decompression of the median nerve (carpal tunnel release) should be undertaken. Unlike in spontaneous carpal tunnel syndrome, surgery is undertaken without awaiting nerve conduction studies as permanent nerve damage may otherwise occur.

**45.** a. This is a displaced supracondylar fracture of the humerus.

b. This fracture should be manipulated into an anatomical or near anatomical position, and this maintained by wire fixation or a plaster cast and sling. Failure to obtain an adequate position will result in severe restriction of elbow movement and deformity around the elbow.

c. The feared problem after supracondylar fractures relates to problems with the brachial artery. This may include actual injury to the artery by the bone end, or compression of the artery due to swelling. Other problems include deformity and late problems with the ulnar nerve (tardy ulnar nerve palsy).

**46.** a. This patient has a malrotated finger. On X-ray you see an anteroposterior view of the MCP joint and an oblique view of the PIP joint. On this occasion it is due to a fracture of the shaft of the proximal phalanx of the finger—it is an indication for active treatment. If it is not corrected the fingers tend to cross on flexion.

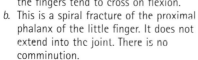

b. This is a spiral fracture of the proximal phalanx of the little finger. It does not extend into the joint. There is no comminution.

c. This fracture was internally fixed to ensure that the malrotation was corrected. Many fractures with malrotation cannot be adequately treated with conservative measures.

**47.** a. This had been treated by plate fixation. This is used to ensure accurate reduction and minimise the risk of restriction of forearm rotation

b. There is a fracture of the radius just distal to the plate.

c. Plates are stiff and protect the bone from stress. This causes osteopenia/localised osteoporosis under the plate and weakens the bone. In addition there is a tendency for stress concentration at a junction between stiff and flexible areas, increasing the risk of fracture at the end of the plate.

**48.** a. The most likely nerve to be injured is the radial nerve in the spiral groove. The important result of this is a wrist drop (weak extensors of wrist and MCP joints), but sensation will be altered over the radial side of the wrist and dorsum of the thumb.

b. Pros-avoid surgery; minimal risk of infection; low tech. Cons—requires vigilant treatment for several months; relatively poor control of fracture position; adjacent joints (here shoulder and elbow) may get very stiff during several months of conservative treatment. Specifically with humerus fractures there is a significant risk of nonunion.

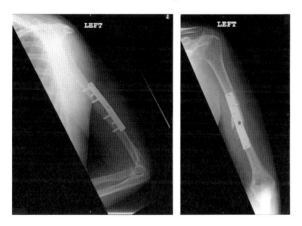

c. Humeral nonunion after fracture in adults is unfortunately quite common. Plate fixation is generally held to be the best treatment, together with bone grafting from the iliac crest.

**49.** a. She has lumbar vertebral compression fracture. In the absence of a history of injury in this age group it is very likely that that this is due to osteoporosis.

b. She should be assessed clinically for neurological change but this is unlikely in the presence of a simple osteoporotic vertebral fracture. If she is found simply to have back pain, she should be advised to mobilise as soon as possible—these fractures are almost always stable.

c. In the absence of any previous history of back pain, no investigations other than simple blood tests are indicated. Unless there is reason to suspect a metastatic fracture, there is no need for further imaging. Osteoporosis in a female patient of this age is virtually certain, and measurement of bone mineral density is not necessary although appropriate osteoporosis treatment should be considered/commenced.

**50.** a. This shows a fracture and partial dislocation of the facet joint of C6. It is difficult to see on the plain X-ray—these must be interpreted with care!

b. There are several methods of managing these fractures, but in general the fracture can be reduced and immobilised for a period to maintain position while the fracture heals, or the spine fused in this position (to prevent future instability). Whatever method is used it is vital to immobilise the fracture site until healing is complete to avoid injury to the cervical cord.

c. Neurological injury at C6-7 is likely to lead to parparesis or paraplegia; there is likely to be some residual function in the upper part of the arms, but impaired use of the hands.

**51.** a. It is not possible to see down to the upper border of T1. This is a common problem due to the shoulders obscuring the cervical spine; further X-rays (or even a CT scan) may be required to 'clear' the cervical spine as the cervicothoracic junction is a frequent site of injury

b. There are fractures of the pubic rami and a fracture of the sacral ala (which is difficult to see).

c. Blood vessels; vagina; bladder. Blood vessel injury and associated severe haemorrhage is a major problem with pelvic fracture but other viscera may also be damaged.

**52.** a. The X-rays show destruction of L1. The history is strongly suggestive of cauda equina syndrome, and this must be the initial provisional diagnosis. The MRI scan (shown) revealed a destructive lesion of L1, which was eventually shown to be myeloma (note that there are multiple other abnormal areas in the vertebrae on MRI).

b. Rapid assessment is important to permit some prospect of preserving neurological function. Cross-sectional imaging (CT or MRI) is required, together with an assessment of likely primary pathology (chest X-ray, breast examination, abdominal (especially renal) ultrasound, full blood count, myeloma screening).

c. Surgical decompression (often with surgical stabilisation of the spine as well) is only likely to halt neurological deterioration rather than reverse it so urgent treatment is important. Radiotherapy can help both pain and again halt neurological deterioration.

**53.** *a.* This is a displaced subcapital fracture. There are risks of development of avascular necrosis and nonunion.

  *b.* The usual treatment for this fracture is by hemiarthroplasty, which involves excision of the fractured femoral head and its replacement with a metallic replacement with a stem down the femoral canal.

  *c.* In a young patient the fracture is treated urgently by internal fixation and decompression of the hip joint (draining the heamarthrosis, which may increase intra-articular pressure). There is still a significant risk of avascular necrosis and nonunion.

**54.** *a.* There is a small abnormality visible in the bone below the fracture. This is a fibrous cortical defect. It is possible that another such defect has acted as a focal point of weakness and precipitated the fracture.

  *b.* Previously, femoral fractures were treated by traction in all age groups. Now femoral fractures in older children are often treated by fixation with flexible nails. This permits more rapid mobilisation.

  *c.* Conservative treatment with traction is usually undertaken in young children. After a period of traction it is often possible to send the patient home in a plaster spica.

**55.** *a.* It is essential to check neurovascular status distal to all fractures. In this case foot pulses should be examined, together with active foot movements and sensation. Pain management is important in fractures—this requires analgesia and splintage (either with a plaster backslab or removable splint).

  *b.* Intra-articular fractures (of which this displaced tibial plateau fracture is a common example) require:
  (i) accurate reduction of the joint surface (to minimise the risk of arthritis and prevent deformity)
  (ii) internal fixation to prevent redisplacement of the fracture
  (iii) early movement of the joint (to prevent stiffness and arthrofibrosis).

**56.** *a.* Tibial fractures can be treated by many methods including plaster, external fixation, plate fixation, and intramedullary nail fixation. For some years the commonest method of fixation of displaced tibial fractures has been intramedullary nail fixation, as this permits solid fixation and early weight bearing with a relatively low risk of infection.

  *b.* Open tibial fractures (and indeed any open fracture) have a much higher risk of infection. Because of this it is usual to avoid large amounts of internal metalwork as this may get infected, and external fixation (shown here) is often used.

  *c.* This history is suspicious of compartment syndrome, and this must be assessed carefully; such patients have: (i) severe pain (and possibly muscular tenderness); (ii) reduction or absence of active toe

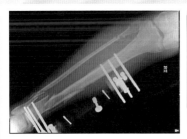 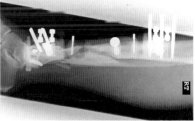

movement; (iii) pain on passive toe movement; and (iv) sensory changes (most commonly in the area of the deep peroneal nerve between toes 1 and 2, as the anterior compartment of the tibial muscles is most frequently affected). Consideration should be given to urgent surgical decompression of the muscles (and if there is doubt this should be performed). In most hospitals it is possible to investigate further by measuring compartment pressures.

**57.** a. Posterior dislocation of the shoulder.
   b. The commonest complication is that this is missed on assessment in A&E. The signs on anteroposterior X-ray are subtle ('light bulb sign'), but obvious on the axial (lateral) X-ray; on clinical examination the humeral head is usually obviously not in the right place!
   c. The dislocation should be reduced. This can often be accomplished under sedation in A&E. In the long term surgery may be required to prevent repeated dislocations.

**58.** a. Immediate swelling after injury indicates swelling due to bleeding (haemarthrosis), but delayed swelling is usually due to effusion. Haemarthrosis often occurs due to an intra-articular fracture or a ligament injury. An effusion in the knee arises due to an excess of synovial fluid and will occur over a period of 12 to 24 hours. Effusions typically occur acutely after meniscal tears.
   b. The MRI scan indicates that she has sustained a medial meniscal tear (arrow).

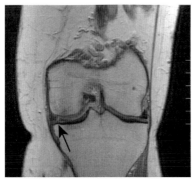 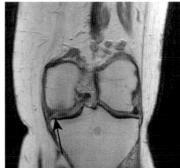

c. Meniscal injuries typically lead to pain, locking (i.e. inability to fully extend the knee) or recurrent giving way of the knee.

**59.** a. This is most likely to be due to slipped capital femoral epiphysis (SCFE). This can be seen on the X-rays. As usual it is most clearly seen on the lateral view and is difficult to see on the anteroposterior view.

b. If the slip is not detected, it may deteriorate. Reduction of the slip is usually not possible, and the epiphysis is pinned in whatever position it is when it presents. A severe slip is associated with an external rotation deformity and shortening of the leg. Osteoarthritis of the hip may eventually occur.

c. SCFE is frequently bilateral (about 20%). Prophylactic pinning of the opposite hip is recommended by some surgeons as a consequence.

**60.** The most likely diagnosis is avascular necrosis (AVN) of the femoral head. Review of the x ray indicates a small amount of sclerosis of the right femoral head; the patient has two major risk factors for AVN—excess alcohol intake and steroid usage. The MRI scans (which are the most useful investigation) confirm the diagnosis, with a large avascular (dark) area in the right femoral head and a small one on the left side as well. A subchondral fracture is already present and is likely to collapse in due course leading to severe osteoarthritis.

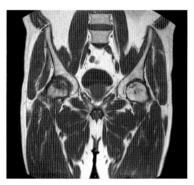 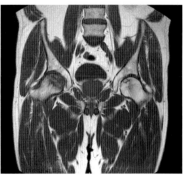

**61.** a. These are known as fracture blisters and are common after ankle and tibial fractures. They are treated expectantly, but are often slow to heal and frequently delay fracture surgery and mobilisation in older patients.

b. This is a bimalleolar ankle fracture. Leaving the ankle in this position is likely to lead to arthritis and deformity, and it is best treated by internal fixation.

c. This is a typical history of complex regional pain syndrome (also termed reflex sympathetic dystrophy, Sudeck's atrophy, or algodystrophy). It is important to recognise this regional condition,

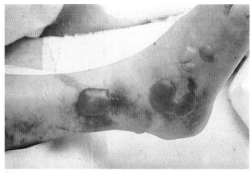

(a)

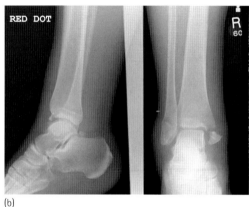

(b)

## 61. This patient has an ankle injury.

a. What are these skin changes and what should be done?
b. What fractures can you see and how should they be treated?
c. Two months later the patient complains of severe burning pain in the foot
and ankle, with paraesthesiae (pins and needles) and intermittent colour
changes in the foot and ankle. What do you think may be causing this?

which typically follows an injury or operation to an extremity. Early recognition is important. Treatment includes physiotherapy and treatment with conventional analgesia (often ineffective) or analgesics suitable for neurogenic pain (amitriptyline, gabapentin). Referral to a specialist pain clinic is often required as persistent CRPS may be extremely difficult to manage.

**62.** a. This patient has a fracture of the pubic ramus on the left. This is usually treated by a brief period of rest and then mobilisation. No surgery is required.

   b. This patient has a low-energy fracture, and it is extremely likely that she has osteoporosis. Assessment of this might include a DEXA scan (to measure bone mineral density). Treatment options include advice about diet, exercise and smoking, and treatment with bisphosphonates (which inhibit osteoclast activity and bone resorption) with calcium and vitamin D.

**63.** a. The patient has an intertrochanteric fracture. Most such fractures require fixation.

   b. The patient is in atrial fibrillation. Most patients with this arrhythmia are treated by (warfarin) anticoagulation to prevent emboli. Re-establishing normal clotting prior to surgery may take several days.

   c. This shows hyponatraemia; it is probably due to inappropriate antidiuretic hormone secretion. Hyponatraemia is common after surgery in the elderly and can cause severe cerebral problems including fits. It is associated with substantial excess mortality. Treatment would be fluid restriction, careful fluid balance (using normal or twice normal saline), stop her bendroflumethiazide, consider a loop diuretic, repeated U&Es estimation, and maintenance of blood pressure.

**64.** a. The pain is very likely coming from the left hip, where there is obvious osteoarthritis on X-ray. Pain from the hip frequently radiates to the knee, and is sometimes more obvious than typical 'hip' pain (which is usually in the groin, thigh, greater trochanter area, buttock, and sacroiliac joint).

   b. Many patients only require analgesia, possibly use of NSAIDs, and a walking stick.

   c. At this age, the only likely surgical treatment is a total hip replacement. This could be a conventional hip replacement (metal stem held in the femur by fast-setting plastic or bone cement; polyethylene acetabular component again held by bone cement) or a resurfacing hip replacement (metal shell to replace the surface of the femoral head and acetabulum). Either one is intended to give good pain relief and is effective at doing this. Risks include infection, thromboembolism, leg length difference, and dislocation. Later, the implants may loosen (aseptic loosening) and require revision.

**65.** *a.* Perthes disease.

    *b.* This would include the late results of a dislocated hip (relatively unlikely) or slipped capital femoral epiphysis or hip sepsis.

    *c.* Conservative treatment would include a shoe raise, a walking stick, analgesia. and physiotherapy. This should be tried before any surgery.

**66.** *a.* This pattern of knee pain (pain (often at the front of the knee) on stairs and kneeling) typically arises in the patellofemoral joint.

    *b.* There is lateral overlap of the patella on the skyline view and irregularity of the femoral trochlea on the lateral view.

    *c.* The mainstay of treatment for this condition is physiotherapy and analgesia. Surgery is often ineffective.

**67.** *a.* This patient has hallux valgus.

    *b.* The initial treatment should be fitting the footwear to the feet, rather than surgical modification of the foot. Only if footwear modification has failed should surgery be considered?

    *c.* Surgery for this condition can be associated with poor correction of deformity, wound infection, nonunion of an osteotomy, venous thromboembolism, complex regional pain syndrome, and even (rarely) amputation. Persistent pain for several months is common.

**68.** *a.* The initial management of patients with multiple injuries is assessment and maintenance of airway, breathing, and circulation.

    *b.* There is severe surgical emphysema and a left pneumothorax (left upper lung edge visible). This patient needs a chest drain.

    *c.* Fractures in patients with multiple injuries should be stabilised to prevent fat emboli, which are a major cause of lung dysfunction after multiple injury. External fixation may be preferred to internal fixation with an open fracture to reduce the risk of bone infection.

**69.** *a.* There is osteoarthritis of the carpometacarpal joint of the thumb.

    *b.* Initial treatment is with analgesia and possibly a splint to limit thumb movement. Local steroid injections to the joint are often helpful. Surgery to excise the trapezium (excision arthroplasty) is sometimes used.

**70.** *a.* There is joint space narrowing, sclerosis of the subchondral bone, and cyst formation. The other typical sign of osteoarthritis (which is the diagnosis) is osteophyte formation—this is not apparent in this patient.

# Index

## T

## U

## V